OCD

Evidence-based Treatments for
Obsessive-compulsive Disorder

*(A Practical Guide to Help Overcome Compulsions
and Obsessions Manage Your Anxiety)*

Rafael Wein

Published By **Elena Holly**

Rafael Wein

All Rights Reserved

Ocd: Evidence-based Treatments for Obsessive-compulsive Disorder (A Practical Guide to Help Overcome Compulsions and Obsessions Manage Your Anxiety)

ISBN   978-1-998927-19-7

No part of this guidebook shall be reproduced in any form without permission in writing from the publisher except in the case of brief quotations embodied in critical articles or reviews.

Legal & Disclaimer

The information contained in this book is not designed to replace or take the place of any form of medicine or professional medical advice. The information in this book has been provided for educational & entertainment purposes only.

The information contained in this book has been compiled from sources deemed reliable, and it is accurate to the best of the Author's knowledge; however, the Author cannot guarantee its accuracy and validity and cannot be held liable for any errors or omissions. Changes are periodically made to this book. You must consult your doctor or get professional medical advice before using any of the suggested remedies, techniques, or information in this book.

Table Of Contents

Chapter 1: Introduction To Obsessive Compulsive Disorder

Obsessive-Compulsive Disorder, greater frequently known as OCD, is a immoderate tension illness wherein a person regularly has intrusive and unwanted obsessional mind, moreover called obsessions.

Obsessions are very horrifying and purpose someone to interact in repeating behaviors or sporting activities to prevent perceived harm and/or worry that earlier obsessions have drawn their interest to. These behaviors encompass maintaining off people, places, or matters and in search of persistent reassurance. Compulsions may also furthermore incorporate internal intellectual counting, examining one's physical elements, or blinking.

Although compulsions in short alleviate the struggling introduced on through using obsessions, this quick comfort only lasts until the following time an obsessive notion or fear is activated. In those instances, compulsive behaviors are regularly executed to help the person revel in "exactly right," with the phrase "revel in" gambling a crucial role. Sometimes, over the years, the compulsions may moreover moreover turn out to be extra of a addiction and the preliminary obsessive anxiety and project were forgotten.

It's important to be conscious that every now and then there may be a smooth hyperlink and motive the various fixation and the compulsion, on the equal time as one of a kind times there may not be any reasoning in any respect.

Obsessive-Compulsive Disorder (OCD) can also take many special bureaucracy, and it truely extends a terrific deal past the acquainted false impression that OCD is exceptional a little little little little bit of excessive hand washing, checking moderate switches, keeping pristine houses, or being a bit bit picky. In reality, if someone has OCD, it will have an impact on some or all elements in their each day life, from time to time becoming so horrifying that it reasons impairment or maybe disablement for hours at a time, each day. OCD is taken into consideration a condition due to this and the severity of its consequences on a person.

Although OCD may be quite excessive, famous lifestyle normally refers to celebrities as having "a touch OCD," ignoring the fact that the "d" in OCD stands for disease. Such remarks in well-known subculture make contributions to the trivialization of OCD and do not anything to appropriately beautify focus. They also are unstable, detrimental, and stigmatizing to people who be afflicted by OCD.

As said within the definition of a sickness, OCD is a state of affairs that interferes with regular bodily or highbrow techniques.

OCD frequently manifests as a hassle and starts offevolved to negatively have an effect on a person's life around past due childhood for men and in their early twenties for girls, but, the contamination can also additionally show up in some youngsters as younger as six. No matter a person's gender, socioeconomic reputation, or cultural records, OCD will effect them. It is currently believed that quite extra ladies than guys have OCD.

It was once the case that sufferers may spend years with out receiving a prognosis, in element due to a lack of know-how of the sickness amongst every the affected person and medical specialists, in addition to in detail because of human beings going to large measures to cowl their signs. Because of the great emotions of embarrassment, remorse, and probable even humiliation associated with what become often called the "hidden sickness," people must conceal signs and symptoms.

The mind and concerns related to advantageous capabilities of OCD, together with unwarranted fears of wounding a cherished one or a child, may additionally moreover frequently appear deeply startling to every patients and non-patients. However, it's miles essential to emphasize that the ones are terrific mind—no longer fantasies or impulsive ideas which will be finished—and that we are able to speak undesired intrusive mind on the subsequent internet web web page.

Most people in all likelihood revel in a few OCD-like signs and symptoms and signs in a few unspecified time inside the destiny of their lives, especially within the course of annoying situations after they provide in to the urge to have interaction in awesome and often unrelated behaviors. For this purpose, we often pay attention the simply unhelpful adage "everybody is a bit bit OCD." Such a term is wildly incorrect even as you take into account that OCD itself may additionally furthermore have a disastrous effect on someone's whole lifestyles, which incorporates their training, employment, and functionality to decorate their careers, similarly to their social lifestyles and interpersonal connections.

When the distressing and undesirable revel in of obsessions and compulsions affects to a extremely good level a person's each day functioning and causes great misery, this represents a important trouble within the medical prognosis of Obsessive-Compulsive Disorder. This is the vital component distinction that distinguishes minor quirks, frequently stated with the useful resource of humans as being "a chunk OCD," from the real sickness.

Recognizing OCD

It's tough to realize what motives someone with obsessive-compulsive disease (OCD) to carry out the vain and repeated behaviors which are a part of the state of affairs, specially for cherished ones. However, it might be useful to attempt to recognize how the problem is maintained to assist us to overcome it or at least make a few sense of it. In specific, it's miles critical to understand:

How it reasons such distress?

First off, allow's be clear that everyone's experience with OCD is precise and complex, and it is not the goal of this internet web page to provide any solutions for any precise character. Instead, we need to depart that to licensed health professionals. Instead, we simplest need to provide a quick summary of the critical factors that guide OCD.

Learning about notions that many OCD sufferers percent is an extremely good region to start:

Inflated obligation is the concept that one is in charge of fending off harm to oneself, a loved one, or others.

Overestimating risk is the concept that some issue is more volatile than it's miles.

Any intrusive mind that an OCD sufferer has regarded quite in all likelihood to go lower back real, and because of their sturdy feeling of responsibility, they feel pressured to take action to prevent it. In exclusive phrases, the two thoughts gas a vicious cycle of compulsive behaviors. The individual with OCD should carry out a compulsion although they believe the amount of chance to be surprisingly low (i.E., there may be little hazard that someone could spoil into my region of employment). This is due to their multiplied feeling of obligation for shielding their place of business.

Regardless of approaches fantastic the effects may be, OCD is endorsed by means of the use of manner of dread. For a person with OCD, the notion of risk is flipped on its head; a hazard of 0.1% seems as probably as a danger of ninety nine.Nine%.

OCD is extensively stimulated with the resource of feelings, and the manner an OCD victim reacts to mind may additionally provide moderate on the supply of those feelings. The scenario that follows demonstrates how various reactions to thoughts effect how we experience and act and can be related to each sufferers and non-patients.

"You're in mattress, it's miles the midnight. A sound comes from the decrease diploma.

It's the dumb cat all over again, you may think, then you definitely definately might probably end up disenchanted and try to pass lower lower returned asleep with the useful resource of the use of burying your head in your pillow.

You have to experience absolutely satisfied and hop faraway from mattress to mention "hi there" at the same time as you pay hobby your partner enter the room due to the reality you have not visible all of them day.

You must anticipate that it's far a burglar, enjoy scared and worried, after which mobile phone the police."

This instance demonstrates how tremendous mind about the identical prevalence also can reason people to experience very amazing feelings (irritated, thrilled, or worried) and behave in quite one-of-a-kind methods.

Consider the spookiest roller coaster you have ever skilled. You are firmly constant, and you are aware which you are secure and stable, however you even though scream and seize the bar tightly as the car slowly lowers you over the cliff as you teeter on its precipice. What makes you afraid and scream out is the "what if" some element goes the incorrect concept. Even in case your mind is telling you which you are ninety nine.9% solid and you are aware that the risk of something horrible taking region is far flung, you despite the fact that scream for a break up second. You can see that even a nice journey must need to be prevented if you have been aware of each minor risk in lifestyles and felt liable for fending off any damage from them. Despite being conscious that they're being too careful, humans with OCD take delivery of as right with they should act "simply in case."

Consider the following situation for a short training workout:

Teaching lecturers typically start via asking the goal market to affirm that announcing or thinking a few thing does not make it occur and that our ideas aren't magical and can't change the course of events. For instance, bear in mind how your lifestyles may also moreover change in case you acquired the lotto does no longer guarantee that you in fact could. The schooling specialist will next ask the organization, which every so often consists of scientific psychologists and psychiatrists with education, to install writing down the call of a loved one after which upload a commentary about some element horrible taking area to them. Despite all the ones surprisingly certified doctors agreeing surely moments in advance that questioning or pronouncing a few detail would not imply it will usually materialize, they may be not often all able to write down the announcement approximately a few thing terrible taking place to their cherished one, or folks who do, then shred that piece of paper into a zillion tiny little pieces.

To higher recognize Obsessive-Compulsive Disorder, the ones examples show key requirements: first, the electricity of a unmarried unwelcome intrusive concept (obsession) to create large ache; and 2d, how such mind may additionally result in apparently absurd compulsions (i.E. Ripping the piece of paper into many shreds).

Anticipate sporting that experience of dread, that feel of risk, that sense of worry with you throughout the day. We believe that virtually thinking about the training workout has left humans a chunk concerned, even only some minutes later. If you may visualize it, attempt multiplying that sensation through one hundred to get a enjoy of what it's miles need to have obsessive-compulsive ailment.

In give up, it is no longer the thoughts themselves that purpose issues; as an alternative, it is how we interpret them inside the first place. OCD treatment is based absolutely totally on this intuitive know-how of the manner our thoughts have an effect on our movements.

However, OCD is an tension ailment, and such mind of worry or risk purpose a great increase in anxiety for the person affected, anxiety that stays excessive. For someone without OCD, it may regardless of the reality that be difficult to truly recognize how an unimportant concept has such electricity over someone, and it isn't always easy to give an explanation for.

I'd need to apprehend in case you, the reader, have ever felt demanding. Have you ever professional continual anxiety? Perhaps you've got professional turbulence on an plane, which motives tension to spike for a time. It does not experience wonderful, does it?

Imagine you are on the lookout for to skip a busy street at the identical time as partially distracted through way of texting to your cellular phone or taking note of tune. You see one factor of the street is clear, so you step into it. Suddenly, you listen a car horn and the screeching of brakes, and your coronary heart begins to race as you recognize you probably did now not look in both suggestions. Your arms begin to sweat, you clench your fingers, and anxiety spreads in a few unspecified time inside the destiny of your complete frame as you see the upcoming car.

Because of your issue, you have been able to understand the hazard, return to the sidewalk, and allow the truck pass without incident—apart from the sweat stain at the again of your shirt. As you skip the street and move in the direction of the sidewalk on the opposite facet because the truck passes, your worry starts offevolved to disappear. Stepping onto the alternative sidewalk reasons your anxiety to proper away go back to normal. You then scold yourself for being a idiot and bypass approximately your day, the tension had vanished completely in a keep in mind of seconds.

Recognize this emotion? Of direction, you do; in any case, who hasn't finished some component similar finally?

This is a regular reaction to a worrying environment; the fear dissipates as the danger recedes. However, for someone with OCD, the problem is that the worry persists; it's far alternatively just like a damaged valve in that the degree of tension does now not short lower. It remains immoderate due to the fact they see the area as being riskier, they experience a outstanding experience of responsibility to prevent some element terrible from taking place, and they often have unwelcome intrusive thoughts that they mistakenly interpret as setting forward a chance. Compulsions additionally preserve someone with OCD from understanding that what they dread may not take region, maximum important them to experience that their behavior turned into really actually worth it when you recall that their worry did not come real. As a stop cease end result, anxiety degrees continue to be immoderate and a vicious loop of mind and compulsions pushed with the useful resource of way of dread and worry is created.

Therefore, anxiety-inducing instances and thoughts bring about awful perceptions of what may want to or might not display up for a person with OCD. Up till a person engages in the compulsion, a protection-looking for behavior, anxiety degrees are excessive even though nothing poor takes vicinity. In extremely good phrases, in place of digging themselves out of a hole, they may be digging that hole deeper on account that the ones terrible interpretations nonetheless exist and the same tension-inducing thoughts notwithstanding the fact that name for further safety-seeking out behaviors.

Another OCD trait is uncertainty; the French used to refer to OCD as "folie du doute," which translates to "insanity of doubt." A person's experience of threat and threat correlates with their degree of anxiety. People are greater terrified of terrible subjects happening and need to be more satisfied that they have completed all they may to avoid them the greater vital the imagined repercussions are. This is the supply of uncertainty in OCD and what motivates many obsessive behaviors. Simply said, OCD can't tolerate grey regions and calls for black-or-white answers (uncertainty)

Let's now examine the two principal factors of OCD:

Obsessions and compulsions are OCD's two key components. The courting among our thoughts (obsessions) and movements (compulsions) while we have OCD is an lousy lot extra complicated, so we can examine it later in this area. For now, this internet web page will interest on defining obsessions.

OBSESSIONS

Obsessions are undesirable thoughts which may be chronic and out of manage for people with OCD, at the same time as they will moreover be persistent pics, urges anxieties, fears, doubts, or a combination of all of those. They are continuously obtrusive, undesired, unsettling, and—most significantly—notably impair the sufferer's capability to carry out each day activities considering the truth that they're so difficult to disregard.

The Latin phrase "obsidere," this means that that that "to besiege," is wherein the term "obsession" originates.

The difficulty is that the OCD sufferer will continually be plagued with the aid of these mind. The time period "obsession" genuinely derives from the Latin verb "obsidere," due to this "to besiege." Naturally, the person that is suffering does now not want or welcome the obsessional thoughts that deliver such severe pain and despair, therefore they'll visit high-quality measures to dam and oppose them. They generally come lower lower returned after a short absence, frequently lasting hours or even days, which also can depart the victim feeling emotionally and physical spent.

Most OCD sufferers are conscious that their obsessional mind are unreasonable, however they no matter the truth that appear very real, and they suppose that sporting out obsessive behaviors is the only manner to eliminate the soreness they produce (which includes avoidance and looking for reassurance). Even on the equal time as there may be no connection amongst their ideals and compulsive conduct, these behaviors are finished to keep away from imagined harm happening to oneself or, more regularly, to a loved one.

It can be tough for people with out OCD to understand what propels a person to have interaction in reputedly absurd behaviors (or anxieties) for lengthy periods. The character without OCD may additionally moreover have the tiniest glimpse into what goes on with a person with OCD and why such absurd behaviors are finished if we were to indicate something horrible taking area to a cherished one, a few aspect so terrible you dare not contemplate such awfulness for even the briefest of moments, then know-how that for someone tormented by OCD such terrible intrusive thoughts plague them continuously for the duration of the day,

It's essential to preserve in thoughts that the ones persistent, non-voluntarily created obsessional thoughts are a trademark of OCD, which presents to the sufferer's discomfort. Regardless in their substance, all obsessional mind frequently reason soreness or an uneasy "feeling." Others surely describe it due to the fact the "feeling" of standard uneasiness, anxiety, and/or pain. Some people say it reasons or will increase worry.

Sometimes, especially at the same time as having intrusive thoughts about violence or sexual interest, a person finds it hard to differentiate among their obsessive thoughts and reality, questioning falsely that truly because of the reality they have got had a idea would now not suggest they intend to act on it.

It's vital to apprehend that some of the most severe obsessive mind—which includes anxieties approximately turning into a pedophile—aren't preceded through real acts of violence or sexuality. We will cover danger evaluation in OCD for health professionals in a later economic spoil.

The thoughts is a robust organ, and in masses of forms of OCD, mainly individuals who center on sexuality-related troubles, it could pressure wonderful areas of our bodies to answer at the same time as we supply hobby to our thoughts, even when we fervently need they might now not. For instance, if we educate you to pay attention to your left foot, odds are that you may don't forget your left foot and enjoy a touch tingling sensation there. Therefore, the ones OCD sufferers whose obsessional scenario is of undertaking incorrect sexual behavior may additionally additionally furthermore discover that their our our our bodies show off physical responses to their genitalia. This is completely herbal and must no longer fear the affected

21

person or the healthcare organisation treating them for this shape of OCD; it just implies that our mind are causing uncontrollable and unpleasant physical sensations. It could no longer signify our sexual orientation or alternatives.

The thoughts and concerns related to OCD can also moreover often seem deeply traumatic to each sufferers and non-sufferers, however it need to be emphasized all once more that they may be honestly mind and are not willfully shaped. They are not each irrational or actionable fantasies or impulses. What is high-quality is that those who have OCD are the least likely to act on such thoughts.

Obsessions and obsessive phobias examples embody:

fearing infection, whether or no longer it's miles in yourself, a few factor, or a person.

being worried about contracting HIV/AIDS or extraordinary illnesses which have received media interest, together with swine or hen flu.

a subject that everything should be located such that it appears and feels in a sure manner (often symmetrically), for the whole lot to sense "simply perfect."

fear of hurting oneself or others physical or sexually.

unwanted and uncomfortable sexual impulses and thoughts, similarly to apprehension about behaving improperly among childs.

worry that a dreadful event can also additionally upward push up.

violence-associated intrusive and unwanted thoughts

Fear that horrible topics will occur if nothing is carried out (at the aspect of that your private home will be damaged into or burned down).

fearing that on the identical time as riding, you can have added on an twist of fate.

You get the unsettling experience which you're geared up to scream profanities in front of others.

COMPULSIONS

When someone has obsessive-compulsive disorder, their herbal response is to combat their undesirable and tension-inducing intrusive thoughts with intentional behaviors and deliberate movements (this consists of each intellectual and bodily actions, searching out reassurance, and avoiding people, locations, and gadgets), the ones behaviors are known as compulsions.

OCD sufferers can also definitely describe compulsions without any easy obsessive fears. In those uncommon situations, both the individual does now not have OCD (the diagnosis of OCD calls for both obsessions and compulsions), or, much more likely, they did as soon as have an obsessive worry or fear but it has for the reason that been forgotten. Their fixation is the uneasy sensation we spoke about at the obsessions web page.

24

Compulsions or compulsive acts are repeated, intentional behaviors that someone feels pushed to participate in via their rigid requirements or in a stereotyped way. Usually, the individual feels a few competition to the act, however that is triumph over via a effective, subjective impulse to preserve it out. The number one purpose of obsessive conduct is frequently to offer (commonly quick) consolation from the tension that the preceding fixation added on.

These behaviors embody repeating first rate acts with a reason in a quite normal and planned recurring, in particular in connection to the obsessional mind frequently completed to prevent imagined chance or harm to oneself or a cherished one.

In sure events, no matter the reality that facts their compulsive behaviors are unreasonable, the individual though feels forced to have interaction in them. According to the data at the preceding web page, oldsters who've OCD-related obsessions and compulsions are the least possibly to act on their mind considering the fact that the ones mind are characterised by way of the use of manner of dread rather than via an purpose to carry out a bit element.

A man or woman with OCD regularly feels a more experience of obligation to perform the neutralizing behavior because of the fact they remember doing so will guard themselves or their cherished ones from harm. Equally, an OCD sufferer may also every now and then have an excessive pressure to discover the best nation for no awesome motive than comfort.

For instance, a well-known and famous stereotype of an OCD compulsion is a person who washes their hands continuously (because of an obsessive fear of infection). When their fingers are grimy, healthy human beings will wash them due to the fact they could "see" that they may be grimy. Contrarily, a person with OCD who's fixated on infection fears will regularly "experience" their arms are dirty and keep washing until they "feel" smooth. Their OCD will persuade them that sporting out the sort of ritual continues their loved ones stable via preventing them from becoming contaminated. The impulse to guard cherished ones and improved feeling of responsibility are what frequently strain OCD sufferers to time and again engage in repetitive behaviors (compulsions)

A compulsion is probably overt (i.E., visible to others), like checking to see whether or not or not a door is locked, or covert (an subconscious intellectual conduct), together with mentally repeating a certain word.

Checking, washing, hoarding, and fine motor motion symmetry are examples of overt compulsions.

The act of doing highbrow in preference to bodily behaviors is known as a covert compulsion, or "cognitive compulsion," in wonderful contexts. Examples encompass mentally counting, obsessive visualizing, and converting scary mind or pix with neutralizing ones. A patient who feels pressured to quietly repeat a series of terms again and again after having a traumatic or violent idea is one of the more concrete times. Or it can be a sufferer's urge to mentally replace terrible terms or pix which could input their cognizance with exquisite ones, inclusive of feeling forced to replace the word "properly" with the word "hell" at the same time as it seems in their thoughts as a idea or a visible picture.

Some OCD sufferers, also referred to as "Pure O" with the useful resource of the OCD network, trust that their most effective compulsions are intrusive mind. People who've "Pure O" OCD wrongly expect that it's miles special from desired OCD and does not have any out of doors compulsive signs. Instead, they anticipate that tension-inducing obsessions handiest stand up inside the head.

However, in reality, a person with "Pure O" will revel in bodily compulsions like checking (numerous styles of checking, from checking on Google to checking for extremely own frame reactions/sensations), searching for comfort from cherished ones or averting unique devices, locations, or humans that set off their obsessive thoughts. The phrase "Pure O" is wrong and useless due to the fact they may be all compulsions (each intellectual or physical). To be clean, "Pure O" is a sort of OCD this is composed of each compulsions and obsessions.

A maximum essential compulsive behavior is a need for commonplace reassurance, specifically whilst the stricken cohabitates. Initially, like every compulsion, while reassurance is offered the sufferer will experience a proper away feeling of remedy, but the uncertainties and uncertainty created by way of the use of the use of OCD will pass once more, and the urge to are looking for greater reassurance follows.

Common times of reassurance trying to find can be to question a cherished one "did I lock the door?", "did I upset or offend you?", "did I flip the taps off?", "did I hit something even as driving?", "did I contact that little one inappropriately?", "did I wash my fingers sufficient?", "do you continue to love me?". Of course, it appears practical for the member of the family to want to assist the character they care approximately feel lots much less annoying and distressed with the useful resource of presenting an answer, but like severa OCD compulsion, wearing out it as quickly as just serves to enhance the desire to retain project reassurance looking for behavior.

Chapter 2: How Ocd Affects A Toddler's Existence

Obsessions and compulsions might start to make it difficult in your youngster to carry out every day obligations, whether they arise together or one after the alternative.

These conduct might also moreover adjust as your child grows older as their attitude on the sector modifications. For example, preschoolers also can have compulsions surrounding food or sleep, but university-age kids may acquire compulsions related to studying. Teenagers, within the meantime, also can have hassle doing their assignments.

But regardless of how the illness offers itself, OCD signs are usually disruptive to a toddler's capability to characteristic.

A psychologist provides, "It takes up some of their time." They find out it hard to hobby on specific sports activities, which encompass circle of relatives, university, and teachers. They can also revel in severe pressure as a give up result.

What Telltale Signs Might Parents Spot?

Obsessions

These are troubling thoughts that preserve crossing my head. A more youthful person with OCD does no longer want to maintain in mind those topics. They believe they cannot prevent, no matter the fact that.

Obsessions is probably detected through using manner of mother and father as extreme anxieties or problems. Children who have OCD may additionally get particularly agitated over:

Things that appearance wrong or out of vicinity whether or now not or no longer terrible thoughts want to come back proper infections, dust, infection, damage, or painful topics that aren't straight away, even, or positioned "simply proper"

Compulsions (Rituals)

A infant could have interaction in the ones actions to experience better. Rituals seem to the child as a way of placing an prevent to thoughts and allaying worries. They appear like a manner of preventing terrible events.

Parents can also see that youngsters:

Unusually touches, faucets, or steps

installation devices over and over and use phrases, terms, or inquiries time and again

having a whole lot of uncertainties and hassle choosing

Clean or wash more than is critical

spend an entire lot of time getting equipped, taking a shower, consuming, and doing homework.

Parents might also additionally want to participate in kid's rituals. Additionally, mother and father may not be aware that anything is a ritual at the begin. For instance, a child with OCD also can want to over and over beg for reassurance. Alternatively, a little one need to call for that a determine communicate or do a little difficulty a exquisite style of times or in a particular manner.

OCD in children and more youthful human beings can also moreover furthermore seem as compulsions, obsessions, or every.

Feelings

Children warfare with OCD symptoms. At first, rituals may additionally moreover seem to provide them with some comfort. But rituals are many. They start to name for more effort and time. Little is left over for children to do sports activities they prefer. OCD sensations, thoughts, and sporting occasions create a stressful comments loop. This also can make it difficult to pay interest in elegance, revel in yourself with friends, go to sleep, or unwind.

Children have emotions like:

When they're not able to carry out a ritual, they experience disturbed, depressed, indignant, worried, and annoyed.

to constantly are in search of parental affirmation that everything is OK

Some youngsters may not disclose to their parents the feelings, anxieties, and actions that OCD creates. They may also cowl their anxiety due to the fact they're puzzled or embarrassed via the use of it. They may additionally moreover take some time to hide their practices. Before their mother and father are aware of it, a few kids can also show off OCD signs and signs for a time.

Chapter 3: What Motives Ocd?

Despite an entire lot of hypotheses and super research, medical docs have now not however been able to pinpoint the precise reason why a person gets obsessive-compulsive illness (OCD).

There are many thoughts, even though, about the probably origins of OCD, which include folks who include one or more of the subsequent: neurological, genetic, located behaviors, pregnancy, environmental variables, or particular events that create the state of affairs in a particular individual at a specific moment.

Below are some summaries of the supplied thoughts, however it is crucial to keep in mind that they are certainly that—concept.

Biological Constraints

Some intellectual fitness specialists have recommended us to do not forget research on thoughts scans and related subjects as proof that OCD has a hereditary or organic foundation. The findings of this study are often described in terms of chemical imbalances within the mind, wrong mind circuitry, or hereditary flaws.

Although it is stated that OCD patients' brains range from the ones of non-patients in awesome approaches, it's miles nonetheless unsure how these variations connect with the proper techniques underlying OCD.

A thoughts test is touchy to diverse styles of mind interest and may, for instance, understand the difference among how the thoughts responds to track being listened to with the resource of skilled musicians and non-musicians.

When a person is irritating in a given scenario, those mind regions grow to be pertinent and "have become on." Therefore, it isn't sudden that there are versions in brain hobby amongst people who have OCD and people who do now not; this does not recommend that OCD is a clinical contamination.

Genetic Variables

Overall, genetic research display that there may be a totally minor heritability of anxiety, despite the reality that a small one.

A member of the family who has OCD or one of the specific ailments on the OCD "spectrum" is more likely to have it than not, consistent with some studies. However, in fact, hundreds of patients do now not even understand one-of-a-kind anxiety troubles or even OCD in their families. Speaking to same twins, in which one will have OCD and the opportunity will no longer have any anxiety troubles the least bit, might solid more doubt on this notion.

This suggests that, if heredity performs a factor the least bit, it could not be the only one, and that, in positive times, received behaviors may moreover make contributions to familial OCD occurrence. Therefore, regardless of the truth that genetics can't be completely unnoticed, it is apparent that it does no longer inform the entire photo and that positioned out or environmental factors may be more important.

In give up, there is no easy benefit to supplying herbal reasons for the beginning area of OCD, specially if doing so reasons folks who revel in it to reduce charge present day-day intellectual remedy options.

Chemical Instability

Mental fitness practitioners regularly use the phrase "biochemical imbalance" to offer an reason for the origins of OCD. These techniques have concentrated on serotonin, a particular neurotransmitter.

Serotonin is the chemical within the brain that communicates between thoughts cells and is thought to have a position in controlling pretty some functions, along side tension, reminiscence, and sleep.

Initially, it have become proposed that there was a intense serotonin deficiency; however, on the identical time as this have end up now not confirmed, a sequence of extra minor anomalies have been placed out, with the general validity of the information very last doubtful at excellent.

The specificity of serotonin reuptake inhibitor (SRI) and selective serotonin reuptake inhibitor (SSRI) medicinal capsules, steady with some professionals, is the maximum powerful proof supporting the serotonin hypothesis. This effect, but, can't be visible as helping the speculation because it was the remark that caused it.

It's vital to be conscious that relapse is extra typically linked to the discontinuation of SSRIs in OCD than in distinctive issues, especially whilst behavioral treatment is absent, which remains no longer in reality understood. This might probably propose that, if no longer as a right away reason, serotonin is a fantastic sized neurotransmitter implicated within the upkeep of OCD.

Overall, SSRIs have a characteristic inside the treatment of OCD, especially in instances of co-morbidity, furnished that the drugs is selected thru the affected person consciously and is used alongside aspect intellectual remedy like CBT.

Psychological Theories

According to further have a examine, a number of behavioral, cognitive, and environmental variables may additionally moreover moreover make a contribution to the development of OCD.

For example, the Learning Theory claims that OCD symptoms and signs rise up from a person learning terrible ideas and behaviors toward previously independent occasions, which may additionally arise as a result of lifestyles sports.

The mental variables that perpetuate OCD had been notably studied, and as a result, Cognitive Behavioural Therapy, an powerful intellectual remedy, has been advanced (CBT).

Learning precept vs Behavioral principle

Researchers documented the powerful behavioral manipulate of sufferers with persistent obsessional neurosis, or OCD, in the 1950s and 1960s. This have become the start of a string of a success case reviews.

This finding and feature a examine ushered in the use of intellectual fashions to deal with obsessions and the introduction of a hit behavioral treatment plans.

According to a subsequent speculation based absolutely totally on this check, ritualistic behaviors are a kind of taught avoidance.

Desensitization strategies carried out in behavior remedy for phobias have been powerful in treating phobic avoidance, however efforts to apply similar strategies to compulsions have failed.

By making sure that compulsions do not get up sooner or later of or in amongst remedy periods, researchers contend that avoidance behaviors need to be actively addressed. This sort of wondering became in advance of cognitive techniques because it emphasized the want of debunking sufferers' expectations of damage at some point of remedy. However, this questioning changed into later visible as incidental to the primary intention of casting off compulsions.

Other researchers created remedy strategies that targeted on publicity to dreaded scenarios at a few stage inside the identical length inside the early Nineteen Seventies.

These many strategies have been in the end combined into a totally a success behavioral treatment software program that used the standards of what is now referred to as publicity and reaction prevention (ERP).

Several studies that supported the use of this method showed that, while a ritual is added approximately, pain and the impulse to ritualize spontaneously disappear while no rituals (compulsions) stand up.

These researchers skillfully mentioned the behavioral idea of OCD, which holds that behavioral remedy for OCD is based totally on the idea that obsessional mind have grown to be related with continual worry thru schooling.

Anxiety is prevented from going away with the useful resource of the avoidance behaviors that sufferers have received (along side compulsive monitoring and cleansing). This leads immediately to the behavioral remedy known as ERP, in which the patient is recommended to avoid avoidance and get away (compulsive) behaviors on the identical time as although being uncovered to stimuli that elicit the obsessional response.

The discovery that the presence of obsessions reasons tension to upward push and that the presence of compulsions causes anxiety to fall became important within the improvement of ERP. People with OCD noticed a herbal decline in anxiety and compulsion goals while the compulsions have been postponed or avoided. Anxiety have become eliminated with in addition exercise. For therapists and sufferers to believe that, within the occasion that they faced their anxieties, issues and discomfort might lessen and in the end vanish, the "spontaneous disintegration experiments" that proved this were critical.

The foundation for next cognitive-behavioral concept and remedy modified into laid by way of method of these early behavioral thoughts and research.

Cognitive principle

According to many cognitive theorists, human beings who've OCD have faux thoughts and growth OCD due to how they interpret intrusive mind.

The cognitive model of OCD states that everybody now and again has intrusive thoughts. However, OCD sufferers frequently have an exaggerated feeling of responsibility and understand those mind as being very vital and crucial, which can also have disastrous effects.

Because intrusive thoughts are regularly misinterpreted, obsessions increase as a stop result. Because the intrusive mind are so frightening, the person motels to compulsive behavior to try and avoid, block, or neutralize the intrusive mind.

The which means that associated with internal (or external) occurrences served as the inspiration for the cognitive-behavioral idea's improvement. Obsessional thinking has its roots in ordinary intrusive cognitions, and right here is wherein the cognitive-behavioral idea draws on behavioral idea. The distinction amongst regular intrusive cognitions and obsessional intrusive cognitions, in step with the cognitive concept, does no longer, however, lie inside the frequency or possibly the (un)controllability of the intrusions themselves, but instead in the interpretation that OCD sufferers offer to the frequency and/or content fabric cloth of the intrusions.

Anxiety might be going to be the emotional response if the assessment focuses on harm or threat. Such assessments of intrusive cognitions and the following temper fluctuations may additionally moreover moreover form a detail of a mood-appraisal downward cycle, but compulsive behavior couldn't be anticipated consequently. Thus, consistent with cognitive-behavioral theories, it's far this interpretation that mediates the ache added on through everyday obsessions through making either their recurrence or their content material material appear for my part relevant and perilous.

Thus, if intrusive cognitions had been appeared as a sign that the person can be, may additionally have been, or might also moreover grow to be answerable for harm or its avoidance, researchers have hypothesized that OCD may additionally upward push up.

The idea of no longer certainly how in all likelihood the cease result is, but additionally how "terrible" this is to the person, is vital to how volatile this assessment is. Additionally, this is going towards the man or woman's notion of the manner they will deal with similar conditions.

Cognitive models claim that the translation of an intrusive perception motives a sequence of intentional and involuntary responses, each of which can also have an effect on how strongly the initial interpretation is thought. Therefore, in OCD, awful opinions may additionally additionally serve as each causative and maintenance shops.

This idea, in step with a few researchers, calls into question the biological concept of OCD because of the fact some human beings may additionally additionally have a organic predisposition to the ailment at beginning but in no manner experience the whole illness, while others can also have the identical predisposition at starting but handiest revel in OCD after gift procedure sufficient gaining knowledge of reports.

Psychoanalytical Theory

The psychoanalytic idea contends that OCD develops because of a person's fixation springing up from unconscious conflicts or ache they skilled in the course of infancy or formative years, or the way a person interacted alongside alongside along with his or her parents inside the route of youth, but it is now a good deal less broadly acquainted than it once changed into. Since the psychoanalytic remedy does not effectively treatment OCD, this idea is currently specially overlooked.

Stress

Environmental variables together with stress and parenting techniques have been associated with OCD, however, there may be presently no proof of this. Although big pressures or stressful life research might in all likelihood hasten the improvement of OCD, strain does now not reason OCD. These, but, are believed to activate OCD in folks which are already prone to the contamination in vicinity of create it.

OCD signs and signs will boom if one unnoticed each day fear and pressure in someone's existence. The frequency and depth of someone's OCD can be extended with the useful resource of issues at work or faculty, strain from checks in university, and common issues that relationships can supply.

Depression

Even in spite of the fact that sadness can also need to, virtually, exacerbate OCD symptoms, the majority of specialists anticipate that melancholy is frequently an impact of OCD in region of its number one motive.

SUMMARY

As you could see, quite some variables had been implicated in the development of OCD, and the proper purpose remains the hassle of severe theoretical debate.

Although severa of the aforementioned hypotheses offer compelling and insightful insights, a combination of the theories can also additionally in the end be discovered to be the proper motive of OCD, and one-of-a-kind elements will probably be at play for every particular character. The reality that obsessive-compulsive illness is a chronic (at times) but mainly curable medical contamination is undisputed, despite the fact that the purpose continues to be being contested through manner of scientists, every so often vehemently.

Chapter 4: Diagnosis Of Ocd

These 4 elements are nearly constantly located in OCD: intrusive thoughts (obsessions) causing anxiety, compulsions (inner or outside, which consist of looking for reassurance or averting unique humans, locations, or devices) causing temporary remedy from the tension, and remedy which could best very last for mins in advance than the following intrusive idea (obsession) takes location. The OCD cycle is useful as it offers a clean illustration of four of the vital additives of OCD, no matter the fact that the real tool of OCD is some distance more complicated and lots less sincere than it appears to be.

OCD cycle

When the nature of the anxieties is eliminated, the aforementioned techniques generally get up, even though in a mainly exceptional manner depending on the shape of OCD.

Most humans absolutely have OCD-like symptoms and signs and symptoms to some extent eventually in their lives, particularly at some point of demanding durations. However, OCD might also have a completely disastrous effect on someone's entire existence, together with their social life, personal relationships, and their capability to have a study, artwork, and decorate their careers.

When the distressing and undesirable enjoy of obsessions and compulsions impacts a considerable stage upon someone's every day functioning, this represents a vital hassle in the medical diagnosis of Obsessive-Compulsive Disorder. This is the important thing distinction that distinguishes minor quirks, often said through using humans as being "a bit OCD," from the real ailment. Although a fitness care organisation will want to undertake an exam to set up a analysis or not, it's miles no longer going that someone has OCD if their character does not reason them to annoying or have a horrible effect on their lives.

Healthcare groups will recall a affected character's diploma of lifestyles impact and the way frightening the signs and symptoms are for them when they ask for help for their OCD. OCD is often diagnosed while signs and symptoms and signs and symptoms and signs closing more than an hour each day.

To decide if someone has OCD;

The affected person ought to admit that the obsessional impulses, thoughts, or visions are a give up result in their minds and aren't the result of every other forces. It need to be admitted that at least one obsession or compulsion is excessive or unjustified. In addition, the obsessions or compulsions must be distressing or notably impair social and/or vocational functioning, frequently thru squandering the affected man or woman's time. Intuition, or the capability to see the absurdity of the obsessions, has traditionally been considered a important thing of OCD. The amount of awareness is significantly various, but, and this is becoming greater referred to. As a prevent end result, some OCD sufferers may additionally furthermore display off normal but low levels of perception, while others can also moreover have belief while now not exposed to a feared situation however lose it while their tension is excessive in conditions associated with their obsessive troubles.

For males and females with OCD, a systematic assessment thru a licensed professional is crucial to get a analysis. The evaluation with a scientific professional will take location over the mobile phone or in person and final for around an hour. To determine if someone has OCD, the healthcare issuer will elicit answers to a sequence of questions, each orally or on office work. Some of these inquiries are as follows:

Do you regularly clean or wash?

Do you frequently check out topics?

Do you have got any mind that preserve bugging you however which you cannot seem to shake?

Do your duties take an prolonged to complete?

Do you fear approximately organizing topics in a nice way or are you without troubles angry with the useful resource of using chaos?

Do those problems state of affairs you?

You have to no longer be concerned if the ones diagnostic descriptions do not in shape what your baby goes thru because OCD covers a massive form of subjects and it isn't always possible to completely cowl they all. The health professionals you spot would possibly understand that the questions listed above are without a doubt a guide and a place to start; an intensive evaluation will embody plenty extra in-depth inquiries about the troubles.

It can be beneficial to prepare an proof of your baby's OCD signs in advance of your assessment in case you revel in that those questions do not correctly offer an reason on your toddler's OCD.

Obsessional signs and symptoms or compulsive behaviors—or each—should be present on the majority of days for at least weeks in a row and be a purpose of pain or trouble with day by day sports for a assessment to be made. The following tendencies ought to be present in the obsessional symptoms and symptoms:

(a) They need to be stated due to the fact the person's thoughts or impulses:

(b) no matter the presence of different mind or moves that the sufferer not resists, at the least one have to no matter the fact that be resisted unsuccessfully;

(c) the act itself should no longer be concept to be interesting (clean relief from anxiety or tension is not seemed as pleasure on this experience); and

(d) the thoughts, photos, or impulses want to be repetitively unpleasant.

A scientific doctor ought to examine you in advance than creating a evaluation.

What OCD isn't always?

As hobby of Obsessive-Compulsive Disorder has improved, so too has the usage of the time period "OCD" to provide an explanation for numerous behaviors that do not have anything to do with the genuine disease.

Obsessive-compulsive disease (OCD) is misunderstood even as the labels "obsessive" and "compulsive" are misused, which moreover minimizes and trivializes the real struggling that the condition can also moreover moreover purpose.

People are increasingly regarding themselves as being "a touch OCD" because the net and social networking websites are applied greater frequently. Obsessive-Compulsive Disorder, which also can surely render a person incapacitated for hours at a time, isn't warranted through the usage of the ones obsessive or compulsive peculiarities, which very last most effective a second and infrequently produce pain or any trouble.

People nowadays appear to need to provide each unusual conduct a call, but once they take a look at with such "obsessive" or "compulsive" conduct as "OCD," they will be not comprehending what it surely is. For example, having obsessions approximately such things as sports activities sports sports, buying, sex, or different a laugh sports activities is pretty one among a kind from having OCD, wherein the person has no pride and the obsessions are over trivial subjects.

OCD moreover has now not a few component to do with people who acquire gadgets out of a particular passion, along with stamps, cash, books with the useful resource of a fave creator, or maybe mementos from sports activities or movies. Collectors just like the quest for and purchase of the artifacts they may be interested in, and they're extraordinarily completely satisfied to speak about or display their collections to others. Hoarders with OCD, however, variety in that they often collect and hoard nugatory, reputedly useless objects out of a fear that doing so may harm them. Hoarders without OCD, instead, are an extended way from pleased or proud.

When used approximately stalkers or "obsessed" fans, along side individuals who are allegedly "obsessed" with a specific character or celebrity, the word "obsession" has additionally come to connote a few issue sinister. Of route, this is definitely unrelated to obsessive-compulsive sickness and does no longer imply that an obsessed person has OCD.

Other examples of compulsive behaviors that aren't related to OCD consist of obsessive mendacity, buying, playing, or intercourse addiction. These behaviors are more often associated with addictive troubles and are known as Impulse Control Disorders. It is essential to keep in thoughts that no matter the reality that all of these may also moreover ultimately motive issues in which the compulsive behaviors cause struggling and pain, the man or woman initially found extremely good entertainment in the interest and there has been no obsession the use of the obsessive addiction. In evaluation, a person with OCD might be inspired to engage in compulsive behaviors by using way of intrusive, unwelcome obsessive thoughts which might be in no manner cushty or agreeable.

While many human beings can also have troubles with a number of the above-noted obsessive and compulsive behaviors and might need specialised help and treatment, they'll be no longer in all likelihood to be identified as OCD-associated problems.

Watch Out for Misdiagnosis

ADHD is now and again fallacious for OCD.

Imagine I'm a 9-three hundred and sixty five days-vintage scholar in a school room. The youngster sitting subsequent to me is coughing and sneezing, and I preserve questioning I'll puke up after school. One day, I get a question to answer to on the board from my trainer. I've been considering the kid sitting subsequent to me and my everyday of vomiting up, so I'm now not certain the manner to answer.

Therefore, the kid does not have a critical attention trouble. Simply stated, it is probably clean for an grownup to don't forget that.

Misdiagnosis is a very crucial trouble. In addition, often, medical doctors have administered the ones psychostimulants to kids who've acquired a false diagnosis. Misdiagnosis and mistreatment are the results.

Chapter 5: Practical Tips For Dad And Mom On The Way To Help A Child With Ocd

If you discovered your kid has OCD:

Discuss your observations together collectively with your baby. Talk kindly, pay attention, and specific your affection. Say some factor suitable for your infant's scenario, such as, "I see you adjusting your socks regularly that permits you to cause them to identical. You're under lots of pressure to reason them to revel in proper."

Let's say that OCD may be in price for the anxiety and the repairing. Tell your infant that a physician's examination can determine if this is the case. Inform your infant that subjects will enhance and that you want to assist them.

Schedule a session with a little one psychologist or psychiatrist. Your toddler's doctor may additionally direct you to the right deliver. They will spend time speaking with you and your teen so you can diagnose OCD.

They will inquire about your little one's signs and symptoms and symptoms to assist them to pick out out OCD signs and signs and signs. If OCD is recognized, they will describe the route of remedy.

Attend your toddler's treatment periods. Discover all of the techniques you could make a contribution. Learn a manner to inspire your infant's development without maintaining off rituals.

Doctors and dad and mom collaborating

Families should be included in treatment considering that parents spend the maximum time with their children. You should anticipate that the clinician will art work carefully with you to offer an purpose for how remedy works and provide homework for both you and your infant to place the abilities they may be learning in treatment into exercise. When a determine or other grownup caretaker attends remedy along their teenager, treatment is satisfactory. They may be able to study the strategies they examine in treatment with their teen and provide everyday aid at the equal time as moreover getting to know a way to teach their child thru OCD symptoms and symptoms.

Learn About OCD for Yourself And Your Child

One of the primary stuff you want to do is teach your self for your kid's infection in case you need to recognize the manner to deal with a infant with OCD at domestic. It can be a lot less complex to plan techniques to assist your teen each at home and outside of it if you have a extra information of the challenges he or she tales. Your child won't benefit in any manner, shape, or shape in case you bury your head inside the sand, act as even though your little one's problems don't exist, or blame yourself for the analysis. The faster you embody it and arm yourself with the information to useful resource your toddler's development, the better. Engage in internet studies, be part of guide companies, discuss with your toddler's physicians and teachers, and examine as lots as you could. A few books to beneficial resource you and your youngster are listed underneath:

Both your own family existence and the life of your baby can be negatively impacted by way of OCD. The urge to perform the rituals in the long run takes effort and time, delaying special, extra critical duties like have a look at and residence duties. Understanding this unique sort of anxiety contamination and its reasons want to be your vital cause. Most children with OCD have a choice for particular items to be in splendid order, and it is able to annoy them within the occasion that they can not discover the order. Your little one might also want to arrange his toys in a powerful association, for instance. He will hold rearranging them within the order he feels is right if you risk to set up them at the equal time as dusting. They furthermore continuously wash their hands due to the fact they're fearful of germs, that could account for this. The majority of childs are unaware they will be repeating conduct. Therefore, if and at the same time as your youngster repeats nice conduct, it's miles your duty as a determine to discover why.

As the initial step in remedy, explaining OCD to kids is important. Putting OCD in a attitude that kids can understand often enables. A therapist may additionally moreover, for example, describe how OCD behaves as a bully. A bully is probably pleased and skip within the occasion that they ask to your lunch cash and also you supply it out of fear. However, the bully will go back the next day to make greater threats considering he is aware about your worry. A bully will call for greater of you the more you cave. OCD operates further. The cause of treatment is to teach a toddler the way to confront his aggressor.

Behavioral and cognitive remedy

A shape of cognitive behavioral remedy (CBT) known as ERP, or exposure and reaction prevention, is the gold-favored treatment for OCD. ERP works thru guiding kids thru the situations that purpose them to nerve-racking in orderly, step-with the useful resource of-step approaches, and a stable setting. With the therapist's help, this permits kids to experience involved and pain with out turning to compulsions. Children learn how to go through their tension through the use of coping with their triggers, and over the years they find out that their tension has diminished.

A little one who is terrified of pollution and germs, for example, would probably work alongside along with his therapist to establish a "worry hierarchy." Together, they could list all the infection conditions he's terrified of, rank them on a scale of zero to ten, and then take on every one one by one until his anxiety dissipates. Beginning with a smooth trigger, like touching clean towels, the kid ought to improvement to more hard ones, like selecting a few component up out of the rubbish.

Therapy must on occasion take vicinity out of doors of the professional surroundings because children frequently show off signs and signs and signs which can be unique to places other than the workplace, collectively with their houses or consuming places. When your toddler has tension in the actual global, your therapist need to offer ERP there. They must moreover ensure that caregivers are privy to a manner to workout ERP outside of training.

Treatment as quickly as regular with week for 12 to fifteen weeks is regularly enough to provide extensive benefits in the majority of mild to immoderate OCD symptoms and signs and symptoms.

Intensive CBT and inpatient care

Weekly or maybe twice-weekly treatment schooling won't be suitable sufficient for children who've considerable symptoms and signs and signs and symptoms and symptoms. If your child's signs and signs and symptoms are drastically affecting their potential to reach school, and preserve wholesome own family and social relationships, and if good sized treatment isn't running, you could want to hold in mind enrolling them in a greater rigorous software program.

Some OCD-specific centers, collectively with the Child Mind Institute, provide immoderate remedy plans that permit children be visible commonly regular with week, condensing treatment and supporting them in making more development more rapid. Children who war with immoderate OCD also can see a change way to those remedies, which often keep them out of the health center.

For youngsters with intense OCD who are not taking benefit of traditional outpatient remedy, an inpatient hospitalization software is each different possibility. A teenager may be recommended to take part in an in depth outpatient software after an inpatient OCD hospitalization to clean his transition far from the recovery putting and help him hold the improvement he has completed.

OCD remedy treatment

Although cognitive behavioral therapy (CBT) is the number one treatment for OCD, children with greater excessive instances are sometimes given each CBT and medicinal drug. Selective serotonin reuptake inhibitors, a family of antidepressants, can be used to reduce a kid's anxiety, which in flip makes the child more receptive to remedy. As the child develops the functionality to control her tension on her very very own, medication can be reduced or stopped altogether.

In sure instances, extra medicinal drugs might be administered to govern immoderate contamination or anger that can be making remedy extra hard.

Make cautious to stick to the desired prescription commands. Never modify your little one's dose without first speakme to the prescribing clinical physician. Inform your little one's scientific medical doctor right away if you enjoy any immoderate issue outcomes or have any questions. Only certified experts may be aware of the effects of solving drug' doses or what can arise if capsules are unexpectedly discontinued.

Related Disorders

Children with OCD may additionally have many issues proper away. Along with OCD, despair, ingesting troubles, and panic contamination are common. It's critical in your youngster to get tailor-made remedy for each highbrow health situation if he has been diagnosed with more than one. For instance, a toddler with OCD will gain from cognitive behavioral remedy however not from remedy for melancholy.

It is critical to take care while diagnosing children to determine whether or no longer they great have obsessive-compulsive sickness, whether or not moreover they have each different disorder, or whether or not or now not they've got an contamination that could appear to be similar to OCD but is a one-of-a-type infection, which encompass acute-onset OCD or a situation at the "obsessive-compulsive spectrum."

The obsessive-compulsive spectrum is a fixed of illnesses with a few similarities to OCD and similar restoration strategies. These problems range from OCD in specific techniques, necessitating professional treatment, irrespective of the reality that they percent certain medical dispositions with OCD and a few specialists assume they will have the identical underlying neurological roots.

It is vital to differentiate OCD from the following ailments that each feature obsessive mind:

Illness tension ailment, in which a little one becomes fixated on the notion that she has a excessive sickness no matter the absence of signs and signs and symptoms, and

Disorder of physical dysmorphia (a infant obsesses on a minor or imagined flaw in her look).

The diploma to which a infant believes her perspectives make a difference. A infant with OCD, for example, can be aware that her obsessions are unreasonable however but enjoy immoderate tension, causing her to experience the want to interact in compulsions. However, a infant who suffers from a problem like infection anxiety sickness or frame dysmorphic disorder can assume her ideals are based totally on fact. Before starting publicity and reaction prevention remedy, youngsters with the ones troubles often require cognitive remedy and techniques to recognize the absurdity of their obsessions. Their tension can even come to be worse through the years in the event that they get ERP in advance than they're intellectually organized for it.

Avoid treating it as ordinary:

OCD is the maximum set up shape of anxiety illness, notwithstanding the reality that we regard it as a "sickness". Because your teen has a compulsive preference, you shouldn't deal with him in a unique manner. Most children can correctly cover their ritualistic conduct until it's far tons later to recognize it. They regularly try to embody their dad and mom in these rituals a very good way to make them appear greater commonplace. They try this because of the reality they regularly understand that it's miles uncommon and revel in the want to correctly normalize their conduct.

Don't offer assurances

Parents ought to analyze the excellent strategies to react to their children without encouraging their OCD because of the truth kids often turn to their mother and father for consolation or help with an obsession or compulsion. Reassurance from a determine may additionally quick alleviate a baby's fear, however over time, it is able to in truth serve to increase the children's uneasiness. Additionally, it without a doubt teaches her that asking her mother and father for help can be beneficial, now not the way to cope on her very own.

Why is it lousy to reassure the child?

Let's suppose I insist on a tremendous method for my mom to say goodnight each night time time. I love you at night time, Mom should say. She should repeat it if there may be any historic beyond noise if the cellular telephone rings, if I do not much like the way it sounds, or if there is each specific interruption. And one time by no means suffices. It in no way stops. Any responsible determine will need to "say it again" and provide that warranty when you recollect that doing so momentarily reduces the kid's fear. However, the children's signs and symptoms preserve to get worse with time. The young infant thinks that depending on Mom to "say it once more" and attractive in rituals are the most effective methods to address worry.

Reassurances are consequently splendid techniques thru which mother and father might also exacerbate a infant's OCD signs and symptoms.

Refrain from accommodating or reinforcing anxieties/fears

Your own family can also have located out to keep away from the usage of terms that your youngster dislikes and to mention "sorry" even as they will be mistakenly spoken. This, however by using danger, moreover feeds the OCD as it prevents the kid from overcoming her fear.

There are several in addition motels. In an try to hold their youngster from encountering sports that could motive anxiety, families could possibly stop traveling on vacations, stop consuming at restaurants or possibly alter their speech patterns. They may additionally additionally need to influence easy of positive names, numbers, sunglasses, and noises that purpose them to demanding.

OCD can be pretty burdensome for families and can critically hinder how households can perform properly. Instead of appearing within the circle of relatives's fantastic pastimes, movements are made to ease fear.

Let's use the following example to demonstrate;

A 12-one year-antique child named Rafe is receiving OCD treatment. Rafe have become worried approximately turning into ill and gaining weight, so he avoided eating whatever that changed into deemed "dangerous," took up to seven showers each day, and averted his brothers and parents due to the fact he belief they were inflamed.

Rafe's mom said, "We hadn't eaten out in months. "He did now not invite any of his friends over. No one from our friend corporation visited us. Our domestic modified proper right into a steady location.

But regardless of Rafe's efforts, his fear continued to govern an developing variety of things of his lifestyles. Rafe's mom recalled how hard it come to be for her family at the height of his OCD. "It changed into pretty tough because it appeared as even though we had out of place our baby. He felt so ensnared through his OCD. He end up out of acquire for us. Spontaneity grow to be now not gift. Even sitting at some point of the table and speaking changed into no longer an opportunity.

Despite the nice intentions of the parents who accommodate their children, own family accommodation is set up to exacerbate the signs and signs. Family folks that accommodate their children are making the signs and symptoms even greater fixed considering tension is sustained thru avoidance.

Rafe's mom stated, "I felt I come to be helping in advance than I learned what inns end up. "When I learned what hotels have been, I modified into devastated. Knowing that I turn out to be supporting the OCD in preference to assisting Rafe horrified me.

The clinician for your youngster need to collaborate with you to discover beneficial strategies for coping with the ones anxieties without traumatic OCD symptoms and signs and symptoms and signs and symptoms.

Developing coping abilities

Through treatment, mother and father have a look at new techniques to react at the same time as their kids get "caught" and the manner to encourage them to apply coping mechanisms or "boss lower returned" their tension in region of asking for their resource. As the kids develop vintage and extra self-reliant, the mother and father must begin to see that fear is not in command in their family.

Siblings and grandparents also can take part in own family hotels, but, they will be frequently not engaged in remedy each day as parents are.

To preserve the peace, grandparents, and siblings can be more inclined to make resorts whilst you don't forget that they may be more of the kid's out of doors environment. In order to prevent them from undermining the remedy, they want to be engaged.

Verify that your toddler's other caretakers use the same philosophy.

For a baby with OCD, it's far critical that they pay interest the equal messages from all in their caregivers, every interior and out of doors of their right now own family. A little one with OCD may additionally additionally end up greater concerned, compelled, and insecure whilst there is inconsistency.

It's a high-quality idea to determine in advance the way you and the other individuals who are responsible for your youngster will react in OCD conditions. For example, you can select to permit a toddler repeat some thing 3 times if your motive is to reduce their repetitive behaviors. This preference need to be finished, and all mother and father or guardians should concur on the repercussions in your baby need to they disobey the law. The toddler can also moreover get careworn and develop a mistrust of the approach if one caregiver is more tolerant than the others. The tool can then malfunction and feed the OCD in place of lessen it because of this inconsistency.

Assist your infant in facing his or her fears.

It is natural to recall that your responsibility as a decide is to reassure, soothe, and instill a feeling of protection in your worried youngster. Of path, you want to comfort and guard a distressed infant and, to the great extent possible, spare her ache. However, seeking to guard a baby with an tension infection like obsessive-compulsive ailment from things that make them stressful would possibly artwork closer to them. You are with the resource of threat tolerating the scenario and allowing it to govern your toddler's lifestyles by the usage of appearing in a normal parental way.

Through treatment, own family people may also moreover moreover teach their youngsters to confront their anxieties in area of run from them. It turns into the determine's obligation to remind the kid of the skills he has located in treatment and to make use of them inside the situation, in area of consoling the kid.

This includes reassuring your little one that he has the inner power to warfare his OCD. Instead of improving his truth, you remind him of the strategies.

The fear hierarchy

A "worry hierarchy" is a tool carried out in remedy in which the child, dad and mom, and therapist paintings collectively to turn out to be aware of all of the dreaded occasions, score them on a scale of 0–10, and deal with them one after the alternative. A child who hates germs and being ill, as an example, might also moreover need to constantly come into touch with "infected" settings and devices until her tension passes and she or he or he's succesful to take part inside the interest. The infant may start with a low-arousal interest, like touching smooth towels, and development to extra tough sports, collectively with maintaining in part ate up meals pulled from the garbage.

Preventing the kid from enticing within the movement that reduces tension is referred to as reaction prevention. A younger man who fears germs could now not wash his fingers after touching the doorknob or the trash, for example. He often involves recognize that his problems are usually unfounded, bearing in mind the development of new expertise. It additionally trains him to place up with ugly feelings.

Limit your participation for your child's rituals

We make a whole lot of attempt to save you dad and mom from taking component of their children's rituals. Therefore, if a infant refuses to open doors because of the fact he is scared of infection, his mother and father should surrender doing so. We do now not want his dad and mom to inform him to prevent or prevent speakme. The word "I recognize that is difficult for you, however in case you war this, you'll grow to be more potent and the OCD will leave" might be suitable.

So the message is, "Hold on, the whole thing can be nicely."

Yes. It's akin to jumping proper right into a freezing pool on a heat day. Your body receives used to the bloodless water within the pool quite speedy if you live in it for a while. We begin simulating this idea at some stage in remedy. You can also save you doing those rituals, and in spite of the truth that you can feel uncomfortable earlier than the entirety, the whole lot can be nicely, we inform a toddler.

Engaging the School

Children regularly show off OCD symptoms and signs in university. It may be beneficial to get your baby's university on board with remedy if that is the case. Helping university personnel individuals recognize OCD is often the first step. Education inside the university is important because of the reality many OCD-associated behaviors is probably compelled for oppositional behavior, academic issues, or different troubles. A toddler's OCD signs, as an instance, can reason him to get distracted, which may mimic Attention Deficit Hyperactivity Disorder (ADHD), or they will reason him to take a totally long term to complete chores and tests, that would mimic a studying problem. Another scholar can spark off his OCD, fundamental to an emotional outburst. Teachers can be extra ready to guide a pupil whilst they're aware of his particular problems and recognise that he is not really being difficult.

The clinician on your child ought to be able to offer particular steerage on a manner to cooperate with the faculty, which includes outlining your toddler's OCD triggers, putting in place a plan for a way the instructor can assist your toddler if he starts offevolved to experience symptoms, and lowering any behavioral troubles or traumatic conditions. Clinicians sometimes visit schools to assist with instructor training at the manner to guide a infant with OCD.

A therapist in your toddler may additionally be able to suggest strategies to assist him or her address analyzing, collectively with non-public checking out rooms and favored seating to lessen distractions or greater time on assessments and papers and using a pc to lessen the outcomes of perfectionism.

Practice at the side of your baby at home.

CBT consists of training outdoor of training lots, which necessitates parental involvement. Children are given "homework" and counseled to hold overcoming their phobias in numerous situations. Family assist and engagement are vital because of the fact exposure and reaction prevention purpose tension and want massive follow-up.

Therefore, you may have a baby that has violent obsessions, inclusive of a male who fears harming his sister. We may additionally try writing, "I will toss my sister down the steps," in a notepad. Then, as homework, he will write this a fantastic type of instances every day. Perhaps we're capable of write it 20 times in a session.

So the concept is that he step by step persuades himself that he won't damage his sister?

He does find out that sincerely believing a few factor does no longer make it real. I suppose I may additionally moreover need to say that I'm a four' 2" antique woman. Is that to say I am? No. It just implies I undergo in mind that. It is probably unsettling to have atypical questioning. But having or now not it is right is lots specific from that.

Parents of a child who fears contamination must urge him to clean up after himself or to emerge as a "human vacuum cleanser," as therapists test with cleaning up little portions of trash off the carpet. In therapy classes, a infant who is fearful of throwing up ought to create a comic approximately "Vomit Man" and practice reading it out to his parents at domestic.

Name the OCD

Give your toddler's OCD a call to useful resource in externalizing it. You might also speak over with it as Mr. Bossy or Mr. Worry. Some younger youngsters similar to the use of their imagination to create unique names. Depending on their OCD situation, some childs call it Mr. Germs or Mr. Numbers.

One approach to reduce the stigma related to OCD is to offer the kid's OCD a call; this gives the child the effect that her anxiety isn't always who she is.

One technique is to mention a few element like this to your infant:

Mr. Bossy is a con man who enjoys bossing you approximately and making you experience stressful. He wishes you to abide with the aid of the usage of his absurd suggestions and live a ways from topics. When you comply collectively with his requests, he enlarges. He could likely annoy you extra as he receives big. When you remodel into Super (insert the decision of your toddler here), you can go up in opposition to Mr. Bossy and defeat him. You weaken him and make him smaller and lots much less effective while you forget about him or disagree together with his absurd suggestions.

Be continual

OCD recuperation is a way. There may be many periods in remedy. Make brilliant you attend every one. Help your infant located the therapist's instructions into exercise. Thank your toddler for attempting. Show out your satisfaction. Remind them that they will be not responsible for his or her OCD.

Your OCD-affected little one will begin thru taking little one steps at the same time as studying to manipulate their worry. For instance, they will only turn on the moderate three instances in preference to 4. So, try to be facts of your infant's development. If your toddler continues to be doing their rituals, withstand criticizing or turning into indignant with them.

Any highbrow health sickness requires time-consuming treatment. The restoration manner isn't quick, and development may be little however everyday. You can also moreover need to sometimes fear that it isn't always functioning.

Even if it would not usually look like it, it is probably top to preserve in mind that via the usage of getting your teenager get CBT from a professional, you're already doing hundreds to help them.

Get assist, then offer it

For households affected by OCD, there are various offerings and assist agencies available. Depending on in which you are, you may test online or ask your toddler's clinical health practitioner.

You can deal higher in case you understand that you're not by myself. You might possibly enjoy hopeful and assured through paying attention to exceptional parents' fulfillment memories.

Since OCD impacts the complete family, some parents find out it beneficial to get counseling for themselves. Believe approximately contacting a therapist if you assume it is able to be beneficial.

Availability for your toddler : Be there

Children with OCD may additionally furthermore experience on my own and alienated because of the fact they frequently have a look at how they range from other youngsters. Knowing that you may concentrate to them on every occasion they want to talk approximately their issues might make your toddler experience less on my own.

Sometimes, children with OCD symptoms enjoy feelings of shame or embarrassment, which can also cause them to withdraw from friends, close down, and prevent asking their teachers or dad and mom for help.

Making an established time to speak in your toddler in a supportive way and concentrate to what they have got to say may be very beneficial. Consider permitting them to apprehend that you've visible positive behavior and that you're continuously there to assist them with out passing judgment or being attentive to them within the occasion that they want to talk about.

Relaxation

Your toddler may additionally furthermore need to strive strategies for muscular rest, mindfulness, or deep respiratory.

You may also practice saying such things as "I can prevent doing this" or "I is probably OK if I do no longer try this" collectively with your infant.

Distraction

You can also furthermore advocate that your teenager engages in some unique interest they select, which include studying a e-book or gambling basketball. Even brief breaks from anxieties might be useful.

A fear field

Your child fills a field with anxieties that they have written down or illustrated. This encourages your toddler to get past their troubles in region of obsessing over them.

A serene setting

This might be a place inner or out of doors wherein your infant may want to have interaction in sports activities to take their thoughts off their troubles.

Create a place that is open, sincere, and alluring. Make advantageous your property is a consistent surroundings just so your toddler may additionally talk in self assurance to you about his or her addictions and compulsions. It may be less difficult for you and his or her recuperation institution to recognize what triggers his or her OCD and the tremendous course of treatment if she or he is more coming near near. OCD can be very preserving apart and lonely for both children and adults, no longer to say terrifying, making it critical now greater than ever that your little one has a space to be themselves.

Set limits

Even even though it hurts to study your youngster in ache, if you do now not create limits, it will likely be more tough for them to conquer their OCD. For instance, if your teenager insists which you dispose of your garments in advance than coming into their room, a appropriate solution is, "I see that you discover this hard, however your OCD is responsible. I'm now not going to dress up before I come into your room."

When you start to constantly set up limits, your youngster may additionally have a "meltdown" or outburst, but they will moreover come to be acclimated to your constancy. Setting limits can finally beneficial useful resource in your toddler's anxiety cut price.

Be stern.

It's critical to be very up in conjunction with your teenager approximately the fact which you could now not allow their OCD dominate their behavior and to act in your terms. Remind your toddler that the purpose is to prevent OCD from taking over their life and the lives of the own family, not to damage or punish them.

Being company consists of carrying through your spoken agreements collectively together with your baby. For instance, in case you tell them that the water may be close off after 10 minutes, accomplish that after the allocated time has handed. Being in advance and then following via is essential.

Recognize and praise your infant for seeking to manipulate their OCD.

OCD is hard to treat, specifically even as it's far greater excessive. It's essential to recognize your toddler for his or her efforts and diligence. One shape of incentive that appears to encourage youngsters to try closer to overcoming their OCD is praise.

Giving reward inside the form of a brief, candy, and easy sentence like, "I'm genuinely glad with what you probably did. You did a superb manner dealing with your OCD ". However, a assertion of this kind simplest wants to be made once. Take cautious no longer to copy the compliments as this may with out issues emerge as too reassuring.

Rewards or reinforcements may inspire kids to stand as much as a number of their OCD tendencies. For example, you could determine that your toddler can get incentives for finishing a certain goal, like washing their hands pleasant as quickly as.

Encourage your infant's self-assurance.

Avoid being too pushy and bringing up each ritual your little one does.

You want to solve an trouble to your youngster as brief as you can. Parents can also become too zealous of their attempts to deal with their infant's OCD because of this. Unfortunately, your teenager is preventing this conflict. Although you may provide advice and manual, you can't exchange this to your teenager. In reality, in case you name hobby to every repetitive interest you observe, you may inadvertently inspire your teen to hold their OCD troubles a secret. Ritualistic conduct can't be stopped in a single day. The first step in the direction of success may be as easy as their know-how it's miles an OCD concept or being capable of speedy cast off workout.

Be trying to find sparkling rituals so you can characteristic as a group.

Children might in all likelihood get defensive approximately their traditions and customs, and they will not want you to just accept any new behaviors or customs. Children frequently emerge as captives to the exercises that offer them brief-time period consolation from their anxiety, in spite of the fact that they do not need to have OCD. So it is vital to appearance out for unusual or unreasonable behavior.

When one OCD dependancy has been eliminated, it's commonplace for each other rule or conduct to take its region. Giving your youngster the equipment to conquer OCD in place of sincerely the particular conduct or rule they're following now might be critical. If you note that your toddler has began out a brand new addiction, calmly talk it with them and assure them that you are there to manual them in overcoming Mr. Bossy.

Adopt OCD Response Strategies:

While terrific rituals are suitable and benign, others may be damaging. Parents need to be aware of which customs are suitable for his or her youngsters to test and which ones want to be discontinued. For instance, it makes feel on your toddler to clean their fingers and feet after roughhousing within the outside. It will help in getting rid of dirt, dirt, and any illnesses. But if he maintains doing it, he can emerge as extra prone to getting a cold and being sick. It moreover topics the manner you engage together along with your infant while he's always washing his palms. You may additionally adopt a more encouraging technique and make the announcement normally in choice to reprimanding him. But be cautious now not to do it all of the time. Your toddler has to learn how to combat this war, and if you constantly nag him approximately it, all he's going to do is secretly do his rituals.

Before you speak, keep in thoughts.

There can be moments at the same time as your feelings get the better of you, and OCD can be very difficult and scary for the complete own family. You ought to be specifically deliberate and attentive within the way you reply in your little one at the ones times. While the rituals your kid does to fight his or her troubles may moreover

moreover seem silly to you, it is crucial to hold in thoughts that such rituals are quite real for your infant. Your child could likely do the whole lot to not have OCD, therefore his or her movements and emotions are not purported to problem you or spoil your day. When you begin to feel irritated, take a five-minute wreck to accumulate yourself. On the instances you do emerge as disenchanted, spend a while talking in your child after you've cooled down so the two of you may provide you with mind on the manner to make sure the identical detail might now not appear once more.

Remind yourself that matters will decorate.

There may be moments while it'll be hard for each of you to control your toddler's OCD.

It's nearly a for the cause that being inflexible and unbending will make subjects worse earlier than they get higher, in particular inside the starting. Your toddler may need to get extra agitated, act out, or have a meltdown. At this point, it is vital to keep consistency and chorus from offering your little one any resorts.

You may be late for paintings, as an example, or your siblings might also argue. It's possibly to try your persistence and once in a while even enrage you.

Nevertheless, try and maintain in mind topics: first, your child is not intentionally disobeying you. They are seeking to manipulate their distress, and their mental fitness difficulty is what makes them seem poor. Second, it's miles natural if you need to have feelings as well. Try to provide a hint mercy to your self, whether or not or not it is because of annoyance, problem, or guilt.

Keep in mind that everybody recovers at a unique tempo.

The diploma of OCD signs and symptoms varies substantially from character to individual. Never forget to gauge your child's growth in opposition to his or her diploma of functioning in place of toward that of others.

You need to push your teenager to carry out on the most diploma feasible; irrespective of the fact that, if the call for to do "flawlessly" exceeds a person's actual capability, it will increase pressure, which causes an boom in signs. Just as there may be a big variety in how intense someone's OCD signs and symptoms and signs and symptoms are, there's a similar range in how quick an individual responds to treatment. Be tolerant. If relapses are to be prevented, slow, ordinary restoration can be finest in the end.

Steer smooth of every day comparisons

During durations of symptomatology, you can pay interest your infant declare that they sense like they're "back at the begin." You also can be comparing your little one's improvement—or lack thereof—to how they behaved in advance than the onset of OCD. Examining sizeable inclinations from the start of treatment is critical. Comparisons made each day are deceptive considering that they do now not take the bigger photo into attention. A mild reminder that "the next day is each distinctive day to try" might probably help your youngster or adolescent keep away from the temptation to turn out to be aware of themselves as "disasters," "imperfect," or "out of manage," that may exacerbate their symptoms.

Reminders of techniques an prolonged manner you've got come due to the fact the worst episode and the begin of remedy can also furthermore make a difference. To have a concrete indicator of increase that you and your toddler can also appearance lower again on, keep in mind using a score scale once in a while. Ask your little one to assess their symptoms and signs and symptoms, for example, using a easy 1–10 scale. You can pose questions like, "How may you price your self at your worst OCD us of a? Since at the identical time as? How are matters in recent times? We ought to revisit this in in keeping with week.

Time by myself is critical.

Family individuals regularly have a natural inclination to consider that they should constantly be there for someone with OCD a very good way to guard them. Family people, OCD patients, or even kids need their personal time, as a result this will be adverse.

Give your teenager or adolescent the message that she or he may be left by myself and that they may deal with themselves now and again with the beneficial useful resource of making age-suitable alternatives about how lots freedom and independence they may be capable of legitimately have. You have other duties and hobbies, and your distinct youngsters and associate probably want your hobby as nicely. OCD can't rule anyone's life. This now not most effective prevents the OCD from resenting you and the rest of the own family. Additionally, it demonstrates to your OCD-affected child or adolescent that lifestyles is a outstanding deal greater than simply fear. Once again, discussing this along aspect your infant's therapist is a exquisite concept.

Everything now revolves round OCD!

Families struggle with the problem of getting discussions which can be "OCD loose," an experience that feels liberating at the same time as attained, whether it's far about inquiring and reassuring the child with OCD or talking about the desperation and fear that the situation brings. We have positioned that considering speakme about fear has been ingrained in own family individuals' minds and is that this kind of sizeable element of their lives, it is often hard for them to end doing so. It's OK to chorus from inquiring approximately your OCD these days. A key element of creating a more ordinary dependancy is placing extraordinary policies on discussing OCD and unique troubles. Additionally, it announces that OCD isn't traditional to govern the residence.

Chapter 6: Exploring Ocd

Outdated Fear

OCD cannot exist with out worry. Fear is OCD's rocket fuel that drives the entire scenario. It is a preventative safety degree that has fairly little use in the advanced 21st century in comparison to the difficult surroundings of our caveman ancestors. For the sake of survival, this robust safety device need to have zero tolerance for failure. One failure can bring about loss of life, consequently one failure is just too many.

Banks protect our credit score rating playing playing cards with multiple layers of safety in the equal way. If 999,999,999 credit rating score card transactions are valid however the one that changed into fraudulent might have been avoided with more protection, this is one too many. If 999,999,999 passengers journey via airports correctly however airport safety drops their defend on one terrorist shoe bomber, this is one too many.

Our worry response want to also bat 1,000. Our ancestors couldn't weigh the pros and cons logically even as figuring out whether or now not or not or now not to seek in a subject wherein lions are stated to prowl, alternatively, they avoided lions the least bit prices! They ought to no longer calculate a chance assessment in their hazard of getting eaten. If they hunted as it need to be ninety nine instances but ended up a lion's supper the one hundredth time, they will had been as lifeless as although they might were eaten the number one time. The effects of their not being capable of offer food for their families or reproduce and preserve their seeds alive would be the same. While today this worry can be counter-powerful, underneath such volatile events, being paranoid and giving into our fears is beneficial for survival.

The motive that is critical is due to the fact putting our fear in perspective gives it a tremendous deal a lot much less power over us. Our minds don't recognise we live in a snug, sheltered surroundings that offers us with the phantasm that meals, water and secure haven are endless resources and wherein real threats to our survival are uncommon.

Have any people ever visible meals or water run out? Has the community McDonald's ever run out of Big Macs? Has the close by grocery keep ever run out of meat or produce? Have our faucets ever stopped flowing with water? It does appear, but how frequently will we discover ourselves without a place to sleep? If we've got got got a fitness emergency, we're able to visit the emergency room and get it dealt with. If there is a threat of violence in the direction of us, we will call the police and are blanketed.

The point is we are in massive component protected from natural threats to our survival. Because our minds are designed to defend us from the ones threats, the machine is out of balance at the same time as the threats do not exist. When actual threats are not present, our minds will discover a replacement and worry some trouble else. In the case of a person that suffers with OCD or perhaps simply tension, threats which is probably lots less large can produce the same fear reaction due to the truth the pampered Western thoughts doesn't apprehend the distinction.

It is definitely certainly worth noting that a tremendous motive zero.33 worldwide nations have a decrease fee of intellectual infection is due to the reality in comparison to us, their minds are inquisitive about survival, the way they'll be designed to be. Our survival-stressed brains want something to fear, so even as real threats are not gift, we blow miniscule threats out of percentage and go to remarkable lengths to defend ourselves from them. The sheer unlikeliness and uncertainty of these micro threats is precisely what lures the worrier into obsession. Threats which can be coming near near which include a massive meteor heading right away to Earth, to the opposite, are a whole lot much less complex for the thoughts to stand. While a catastrophic meteor is not any doubt horrifying, it isn't always complex. The meteor is coming and there can be nothing you can do about it (even though Bruce Willis would possibly in all likelihood beg to differ), so a victim's mind may not be thrust into an internet of obsession.

Along with mastering right reasoning, locating processes to reduce worry is paramount in the journey to restoration. Being aware about why our minds behave the manner they do can pass an prolonged manner. We can not consciously command our worry to head away due to the reality this is like pouring grease on a fireplace; it will simplest make it more potent. Truly being glad that what we fear isn't always the forestall of the sector fights again at the deliver and gives us greater power over the extra primitive, vintage elements of our minds in desire to letting our minds manipulate us.

Chapter 7: Thumb In Front Of The Mind

To gain angle of approaches thoughts and doubts can appear to us a good buy bigger than they surely are, a visible is vital. If willing, I'd need to invite the reader to walk outside at night time and reflect onconsideration on the moon. Then, stick your thumb within the front of taken into consideration one of your eyes and close the alternative. What seems large, your thumb, or the moon? Even despite the fact that the distinction in size is exponential, even as positioned inside the vantage issue of covering maximum of your vision, a few factor as tiny as your thumb can without a doubt appear huge than a few problem as large because the moon.

Our mind, fears and doubts are commonly small, however they appear good sized to us because of the reality like a thumb blockading our eyes from view, mind can block our minds from view. The human beings close to us can have a look at that that is happening because of the reality they don't have a concept blocking their vision of the a whole lot huge photo of our lives.

The key takeaway then is to be aware of this trick that our brains play on us. When a idea feels overwhelmingly massive, preserve in mind the thumb in the the front of the eye. Objects inside the front of the mind won't be as massive as they seem.

Is OCD Solely Faulty Wiring of the Brain?

This is likely the subject that requires the maximum rationalization because it ties the whole technique together. This isn't a scientific or medical ebook this is based mostly on posted studies, so I will stick strictly to the individual of doubt and the reasoning that surrounds it.

Far too many therapists tell OCD sufferers that their obsessive thoughts and doubts are irrational. Many of those therapists are satisfied that OCD and different anxiety issues are altogether irrational. This is over-simplified, stupid, or even dangerous. "It's absolutely your OCD" is a not unusual exceptional affirmation. What is ironic at the floor right here is that brushing off and correcting doubts on this sort of manner contradicts the fundamental tenants of Exposure and Response Prevention Therapy (ERP), OCD's flagship treatment. This aspect might be mentioned further in a few exceptional bankruptcy.

The reality then, much like most topics in life, isn't black or white. Every doubt has an element of legitimacy and is in no manner simply irrational. Do even the maximum excessive OCD sufferers doubt that the sky is blue? No, because they might bypass outside and observe it as blue. Do they doubt the Theory of Gravity? No, because of the reality if they jump, they arrive back down. Do they doubt that water makes them moist? No, because of the truth they recognize what occurs when they shower each night time time time (with a bit of luck). The list is going on and on, but without a doubt, obsessive minds are capable of identifying and being at peace with absolute truth, so it is not sensible to signify that OCD patients are incapable of embracing truth due to their mind chemistry.

Further proof that OCD can honestly be rational is that sufferers, specifically in simple phrases obsessive sufferers, can enjoy signs and symptoms and signs and symptoms and signs and symptoms while on each facets of a fence. A individual can revel in obsessive doubts about their beliefs as a Democrat, after which revel in similar doubts in a while in existence with contradictory ideals as a Republican. A Christian can enjoy obsessive doubts about their faith, then adopt a contradictory ideology as an Atheist and however experience comparable doubts. This is what came about to me.

I spent years as a spiritual Christian and continued excellent doubts observed through the use of infinite what ifs and logical loopholes, but then professional the same doubts, what ifs and logical loop holes as soon as I actually have become an agnostic. I believed at one component in my existence that Jesus physical rose from the useless, and later in lifestyles am satisfied that the resurrection became a spiritual enjoy. Even even though I sincerely have expert doubts with each ideals, they may be contradictory and can't every be proper. One of them is proper and certainly one of them is wrong. So, if OCD can be present on each aspects of a fence, then certainly it is feasible for OCD doubt to be wrong, as we recognise, but additionally possible for it to persuade us towards truth.

Since every doubt has at least a few valid cause for contemporary, does that imply that each doubt is one hundred% accurate? Of path now not! A doubt having some legitimacy is not the same as it being actual. OCD sufferers aren't goal with their fears, in order that they count on worst case conditions and catastrophize. For instance, a sufferer who compulsively washes her fingers can also count on she will die if she doesn't wash her hands one hundred times in an afternoon. This is maximum likely fake, however there may be at the least a few validity to the worry due to the fact it's far at the least feasible to die from germs. Someone who fears they'll damage a cherished one most probable will not do it, however the fear has at the least some valid cause for present because of the reality the sufferer is bodily able to such an act and can in reality have a valid reason to be upset with that man or woman.

So, if OCD may be every rational and irrational, how are we in a role to tell the difference? I will endorse that when we will discover a place wherein our aware minds are in concord with our unconscious, extra instinctual minds, then we are on the right song. This is how I overcame my situation. I did not run far from my doubts and disregard them as honestly being my OCD speakme. I stared them in the face, belief them via and located ideals I may be at peace with. The trap is that doing so nearly killed me. I needed to truly adjust my existence and my idea styles to get to in which I had to be, and this is in which many patients get stuck. Truly addressing the idea motive of your OCD and overcoming the state of affairs includes being brutally honest with yourself. Your self-discovery may want to even reason leaving, or at least notably altering your mindset of a interest, a marriage or perhaps a faith. These are massive life adjustments and aren't clean, but can be what is crucial for recovery.

Traditional OCD vs. Pure Obsessional OCD

When maximum humans remember OCD, they think about the conventional examples consisting of a victim washing his palms repetitively. What many don't realise is that OCD also can take area absolutely in the mind, so as that in choice to acting physical rituals like washing one's fingers, sufferers perform repetitive thoughts, affirmations and super mental rituals to steer themselves that the doubts are not real. Even despite the fact that you can't check the rituals, the state of affairs is still very a good buy as actual. In truth, the certainly obsessional model of OCD is frequently extra extreme due to the fact the awful outcomes of what's being feared can be worse than those of conventional OCD. For instance, the outcomes of committing the unforgivable sin are a long way greater excessive than leaving your doorways unlocked. Spending an eternity in hell is an awful lot more frightening than your house being robbed.

Now, whilst you hold in mind that mental and physical rituals function the identical manner within the mind, it's miles simplest herbal to expect that patients can enjoy each conventional and Pure Obsessional OCD in a few unspecified time in the destiny of their lives, or perhaps on the same time. My number one situation is Pure O, but as long as I can consider, I also have struggled with outward obsessions together with checking my cellular telephone or alarm clock time and again or repeating notable phrases and phrases. From what I actually have additionally seen in fellow sufferers, this is the norm in vicinity of the exception.

The connection among the 2 kinds of OCD may be very essential, now not so much as to initiate a dialogue of treatment, however due to the truth Pure Obsessional OCD is instead misunderstood and lacks hobby. In well-known, highbrow fitness is centuries at the back of physical fitness due to the reality the body is a whole lot much less complicated to check than the mind. Purely Obsessional OCD is therefore a brilliant deal more difficult to apprehend, diagnose and cope with than Traditional OCD. Pure O sufferers conflict to discover records and assist from their own family, buddies or maybe their therapists. Suffering from this type of situation is tough enough, so struggling on my own is even greater of an uphill war.

Chapter 8: The Problem With Labeling

Labeling intellectual illnesses may be a sloppy mess. It is also now and again vain and might do more harm than specific to a victim. There are some motives for this:

First, many illnesses indexed within the DSM are exaggerations of normal human stories. Take the big two, tension and depression, for instance: Everyone gets disturbing at instances and reviews at the least mild melancholy in the end of their lives. These human evaluations are as herbal as hunger, thirst, drowsiness and sexual desire. Similarly, everyone furthermore research obsessive mind and performs rituals to reduce the anxiety. These research are handiest labeled a disease once they intervene with ordinary life, it is subjective to a degree. These situations can be advanced via the use of any wholesome person the equal way each person can emerge as overweight in the event that they eat now not a few thing however ice cream and live a sedentary way of life.

The different essential challenge of labeling psychiatric issues is that plenty of them overlap. Obsessive thoughts are a commonplace symptom of melancholy, and despair is a not unusual symptom of OCD. So, what comes first? The melancholy, or the obsessions? The chook, or the egg? What is the right label? Is it despair with corresponding obsessive thoughts, or obsessive thoughts with corresponding depression? Do you normally deal with the depression, or the OCD? These are the sorts of knots that therapists and psychiatrists regularly discover themselves in.

Clearly, common highbrow troubles are particularly tough to label. In addition, at the same time as labeling is essential for treatment, it frequently has negative effects which include producing a horrific stigma that society projects upon patients, and/or that patients venture upon themselves. People who are categorized as having OCD may also promote themselves short and experience no longer so proper as the rest of society while people with the equal symptoms and symptoms, however who have never been labeled mentally sick with the aid of way of a professional, can accumulate plenty greater due to the fact they do not see themselves as top notch. They don't make the equal excuses.

Imagine someone this is genetically inferior in duration and physical electricity. Is it better for him to label himself as a willing individual, rely himself out as super and avoid bodily hobby, or, is it better for him to widely recognized his inherent downside, however counteract it with the useful resource of the usage of hitting the fitness center every day to overcome it and gather his energy to a degree that gives him self assurance? One belief is without a doubt one among defeat and victimization, on the identical time as the alternative is taken into consideration genuinely one in every of self-empowerment. The latter will yield higher consequences every time.

The Not So Safe Safe Approach

As cited above, the popularity quo notion of OCD is that it's far irrational. However, cognitive remedy for OCD involves SLOWLY desensitizing a victim to the horrifying stimulus, so a therapist have to no longer inform a compulsive hand washing machine, "It's in reality your irrational OCD and also you're no longer going to get sick. Don't fear about it." That wouldn't artwork! The technique is the opposite of the way you're speculated to address OCD. Why then do therapists try and dismiss the entire infection as faulty wiring of the thoughts? Why teach a effective treatment (ERP), and then provide counseling this is contradictory to that treatment?

It is a extremely good dichotomy indeed no longer great because of the truth many, if no longer most professionals contradict their very very very own remedy with reassurance, but additionally because of the truth the idea is so clean that it shouldn't be neglected. It amazed me in my personal adventure, and helping distinct OCD sufferers, how regularly this occurs and the manner regularly therapists and exceptional professionals get it wrong. I acquire as proper with the cause it is unnoticed is because of the nurturing surroundings of a scientific placing that strives to comfort a sufferer. Unfortunately, quick consolation is OCD's satan disguised as an angel similar to the quick restore of any addiction. When a therapist comforts a victim and over and over assures her or him that the whole thing is proper sufficient, the therapist then really assumes the function of acting compulsive rituals. While the therapist's intentions are natural, she is doing no longer anything extra than feeding the sufferer's addiction and retaining the cycle going. In this case, rather than appearing rituals in private, the victim in reality performs rituals with the therapist as an alternative.

Treatment for any highbrow or physical infection ought to encompass techniques validated by way of empirical proof. This is the way it must be and the manner it commonly may be. There is not any cash in the treatment notwithstanding the reality that. Sometimes ripping off a band resource makes a wound worse earlier than it gets higher, and on occasion ripping off this band useful useful resource outcomes in a disastrous very last consequences. So, the hazard (s) of the real treatment for OCD, which I agree with to be correcting faulty wondering, leads maximum specialists to take the secure route and use Cognitive Behavioral Therapy collectively with ERP with little threat for catastrophe. The turn facet is that a consistent treatment with a decrease threat for disaster also has a lower ceiling for fulfillment. Conventional therapy is low threat, low reward at the equal time as gutting out the inspiration trouble of defective thinking is immoderate risk, high reward.

The Limits of Exposure and Response Prevention Therapy

Exposure and Response Prevention, OCD's treatment of preference, will increase intellectual flexibility with the beneficial resource of often exposing the sufferer to the horrifying stimulus in order that they become a bargain an awful lot much less and less sensitive to it, which in the end reduces the anxiety. If a sufferer fears germs and washes his palms 100 times a day, ERP will guide him to clean his arms 90 times a day one week, then 80 the following, 70 the following and so forth until he receives all the way down to a wholesome 10 times a day.

Is this clearly the best method despite the fact that? It can be insightful to observe the signs and signs and signs and symptoms and signs and remedy of OCD to the ones of a mosquito chew. When you're bit via manner of the use of a mosquito, it leaves a lump that itches. Scratching it makes it experience higher for a short time body, but then the itch becomes even more immoderate next time. This stronger itch requires a more potent scratch which sneaks into a vicious cycle: The extra it itches, the greater you scratch, and the more you scratch, the more it itches. Drug addiction works the same way: The stronger the cravings, the bigger hit of medicine is important, and the larger hit of medication, the more potent the cravings might be. OCD isn't any extraordinary with intellectual and overt compulsive rituals, but unlike a mosquito chunk, the itch to act compulsively and obsess does now not heal itself biologically and depart through the years. As I preserve to pressure as nicely, treating the signs and symptoms and signs by myself does now not clearly paintings either.

Let's evaluate the two scenarios element via aspect and surely task in context the perception that ERP Therapy is the first-rate method to treat OCD. How ought to ERP characteristic in treating a mosquito chew? The sufferer should frequently scratch the location a lot less and less. Yes, this will make the itch skip down, however it wouldn't make it depart, and it without a doubt might not save you bites in the future. The actual remedy is to area on insect repellant or avoid going out into the woods at night time time time to avoid mosquitos altogether.

No medical doctor will inform someone this is concerned about mosquito bites that the outstanding remedy for them is to now not scratch the itch; the fine treatment is to keep away from bites within the first location. So, why are we able to have an notable time scratch prevention due to the fact the first-rate treatment for OCD? Why do we not train a manner to save you and treatment it? As touched on above, healthcare professionals desiring to cowl their very very very own asses and being blind to the muse (s) of the condition, further to political correctness, are primary elements. If a therapist tells a person suffering from immoderate fear that he or she might be homosexual to check the waters and sleep with a member of the identical intercourse, the therapist is probably breaking every rule within the e-book in addition to be reliable if this behavior effects inside the harm of, or on behalf of the consumer. Even although this advice might be cheap, a therapist is probably now not able to offer it due to legal responsibility.

I in reality have moreover decided that this treatment satisfactory appears to be effective if the obsession is irrational because of the fact our minds are very difficult to trick. If your mind is happy that a few issue it fears is a actual threat, it's far near not possible to persuade it in any other case, so sheer scratch prevention will now not be powerful and will even make it worse. Consider a sufferer that fears he's going to die in a car crash if he drives at the motorway. This is most in all likelihood fake and his unconscious thoughts is aware about it, so the slow desensitization of ERP is probably pretty powerful. To the opposite, a sufferer that is uncertain about his sexual orientation ought to have a much extra tough time education his thoughts to allow it waft. He's going to want to decide it out ultimately and be at peace collectively together along with his state of affairs, so warding off scratching the itch to obsess over his sexuality will only cast off the considering, that may come once more later with a vengeance. In situations like this even as dealing with signs and symptoms and signs and symptoms does not produce lasting development, turning into a higher logician is the simplest way.

In brief, sufferers can not depend on a therapist that is handcuffed with the useful useful resource of scientific restraints and lack of know-how of their condition to provide a remedy. Sufferers want to dig deep and discover it themselves.

I cannot stress sufficient that there can be no substitute for addressing the inspiration of a hassle. Medication and Cognitive Behavioral Therapy consisting of ERP aren't the quality remedy plans for OCD due to the fact they in reality treat the signs and symptoms. Rather, correcting the defective wondering that caused the OCD within the first region want to be first and maximum crucial. If corresponding remedy can assist alongside the manner, it need to be used of course, however it can't be the number one attention. We need to correct faulty questioning. Sometimes truly being aware of the pitfalls in reasoning may be a big assist, but if a complete path correction in notion or a life-style trade is essential, the overactive and frequently greater modern OCD-inclined thoughts is in fact able to finding a way.

Chapter 9: Constructive Obsessing

Everyone obsesses, and everybody performs repetitive rituals to reduce anxiety. It is not an all-or-not whatever scenario wherein OCD sufferers do, and "regular" people do now not. OCD sufferers in fact exercise this behavior MORE than everyone else. As cited previously, labeling OCD patients as mentally unwell can restrict the scope wherein the abnormality may be corrected, or re-directed to greater positive behavior. Since we've already considered the bounds of lowering signs and signs and symptoms, we ought to in addition hold an open thoughts to greater revolutionary approaches of combating the contamination.

Let's task off a piece and do a little comparing: If you personal a domestic dog Tiger, do you educate it to now not be a Tiger? Or, do you boost it in a habitat and feed it meals that allows the Tiger to stay more cautiously to its right nature? Do we educate our puppies to be cats? If we had been to undertake definitely certainly one of our relative chimpanzees, would in all likelihood we raise it much like our unique kids?

Resisting an animal's authentic nature may not be well-suggested, so we have to be cautious about doing so with humans. Thankfully in a loose society, we have endless profession opportunities that permit humans to top notch express who they may be. Creative people can play tune and create art. Detail-orientated humans can be accountants. Sexually-deviant human beings can paintings in grownup entertainment. Passionate those who need to argue can end up legal experts. People who are driven thru intensity can art work in regulation enforcement, within the navy or play contact sports activities activities sports activities.

When we connect the dots, we should come to the natural end that searching out to educate an obsessive thoughts now not to obsess might not be the first-class technique. I located as my scenario advanced that my obsessive nature although carried on, however in lots much less unfavourable approaches. Rather than obsessing over subjects that triggered me intellectual distress, I positioned myself obsessing over food, sports activities, politics, social media and courting. I decided out that OCD is not constrained to my primary troubles; my obsessive nature can rub off in all regions of my lifestyles.

One strategy I honestly have consequently determined very powerful is to redirect my marathon interest to more powerful conduct along with exercise, writing, playing music, carrying out dreams at paintings and doing superb subjects for my family and pals. I am in a function to carry out greater in those quests than the average man or woman because of my unusual abilities to consciousness for lengthy periods of time, count on creatively and express large quantities of affection and passion. Even the struggling I continued may be used as a incredible as it has allowed me to amplify enormously thick skin and uncharted perseverance. Since I am going to be the equal passionate, obsessive, meticulous bastard regardless, I might also as well be one which affords cost to the location.

In addition, modern-day psychology is likewise a very current phenomenon. Before the last few hundred years, humans with fantastic thoughts chemistry were not categorized mentally sick the manner they may be now. Great leaders and influential minds that might be considered mentally sick in recent times had been heroes within the historic worldwide. Jesus and Buddha are amazing examples as ruminating in the barren place looking for truth for weeks at a time is a textbook display of Pure Obsessional OCD. These people concept in a one-of-a-type way and challenged the repute quo. They had been discovered and favored whereas nowadays, such humans is probably put on treatment and managed by means of the usage of society out of fear of the stigma carried through the use of their label (s). Musicians, artists, inventors and extraordinary proficient human beings have a colorful track record of intellectual turmoil due to the fact the same parts of their minds that make them especially capable furthermore depart them susceptible to being unstable.

What it boils proper right down to is OCD sufferers want no longer succumb to the message given to them with the useful resource of society that by way of hook or by means of criminal regular interprets to inferior or unworthy. People who own the brainpower to drown of their very very own mind can make a contribution to the world in remarkable strategies if their competencies are channeled efficiently and inside the occasion that they get out of their very own manner. It is as tons as you, the reader, to find out your path to try this, but discover your path you have to!

Common OCD Themes in Perspective

In this segment, I would love to discover most of the maximum common issue subjects, or triggers, for OCD and the manner faulty wondering contributes to them. The handiest ones that I surely have substantial private revel in with are non secular and relationship OCD, so there will sincerely be a gap in having the ability to narrate to the others. I am now not trying to solve all of them single-handedly. As stated formerly, the purpose is to open new doorways for you as a way to start you down a course of expertise the way to address the muse of your situation. There is not any such element as a brief restore to any immoderate hassle, and this approach isn't any exception. This is honestly purported to be a place to start, so start we can!

Hand Washing/Fear of Germs

Many people experience that it's miles unacceptable to be ill. Do any people truely understand everybody that struggles with this intrusive worry that did not growth up in a wonderful steady surroundings wherein their dad and mom and teachers went out in their manner to maintain them easy and healthy?

I'm wonderful they exist, but I really have no longer met any. In my private revel in, no matter the reality that I am fairly susceptible to tension and obsessive behavior, I actually have in no manner had an exaggerated fear of germs due to the truth I grew up in the South wherein I come to be outside playing within the woods and in the dust every weekend. Like many disconnects from our herbal ecosystems, the urge to stay clean and wreck free the actual worldwide complete of sickness and sickness can be overwhelming to individuals who are taught at a younger age that contamination is a tragedy.

The fact: Common regular germs will not often make you sick, and when they do, it's commonly now not a large deal. We are to be had in contact with infinite germs each day. Most micro organism are useful and lots of even live indoors oldsters. Most viruses are without difficulty destroyed via our immune structures. There are viruses that do hundreds of proper, which consist of a few that would even be capable of treatment amazing styles of most cancers. Our ancestors survived for tens of tens of millions of years with out present day hygiene and had been far much more likely to get eaten via the usage of a predator or murdered with the aid of a rival than killed through some component just like the commonplace cold, so our refuge from the previous reasons an exaggerated fear of the latter. Even if we do get ill and pass on, the universe will still preserve on simply exquisite with out us.

In short, probable the best antidote to the obsessive compulsions of germ cleaning is to persuade oneself on a deep, unconscious diploma that germs are not that volatile. This is in essence what ERP therapy does via motion, however altered notion is an prolonged manner extra effective and the motion will certainly have a have a look at.

Checking

In each different example of the incompatibility of our primitive minds developed over thousands and hundreds of years designed to stay on being thrust proper into a modern-day, cushty worldwide, our environment now not being sincerely so as is one extra difficulty this is all too clean to worry.

While our over-touchy brains labored nicely to combat off hunger, contamination and predators for our ancestors, from time to time a door left unlocked or a variety left on may be the best danger a present day man or woman faces. This hyperbolic sensitivity to such insignificant threats is difficult to unlearn, but no longer impossible. Ideally, we might have all spent the number one 18 years of our lives in a 3rd global u . S . A . Learning to take no longer something with no consideration, and then moved to paradise in a evolved united states of the united states of the usa. We might be able to see that unlocked doors aren't that big of a deal in the grand scheme of things. Since that isn't always viable, likely the following first-rate issue is to alter our perspective as a result.

Chapter 10: Harm Ocd

A very short time inside the past in an evolutionary timeline, we lived as savages. We competed with every unique for meals, intercourse and steady haven. We fought and killed even as crucial. These savage instincts advanced over masses of hundreds of years whilst the modern-day, Western mind-set that suppresses our preference to violently compete advanced in only a few hundred. Our minds in reality have no longer had sufficient time to comply, and the two techniques of thinking often are to be had war with each distinctive. We are competitive beings and may in no way live as completely altruistic humans. We still compete, however rather than compete with violence, we compete with every one-of-a-kind in organization, politics, instructors, athletics and peer bonding.

The humans I virtually have talked to that conflict with this topic commonly have been raised in a strict non secular or special strong environment wherein they were taught the fable that all existence is sacred to the quantity that there can be in no manner the appropriate time for life to be lessen brief or for evil to be punished. This ideology is basically incompatible with our herbal fight for survival and is a incredible instance of the way cutting-edge society can disconnect our minds from reality.

What appears to arise with these sufferers is any proposal of violence is a purpose for misery. They enjoy obligated to distance their natural enchantment to violence from their identity as parents which is probably morally superior to it. The sufferers then set their minds in a loop of searching for to steer themselves that they may be now not capable of violent acts, often escalating to weird, intrusive thoughts in conjunction with harming harmless cherished ones. In such times, it's nearly similar to the suppressed thoughts fights decrease returned through announcing, "Oh yea? You don't suppose you're able to violent acts? Watch this photograph of you doing so time and again over again till you face fact."

I am in no manner encouraging everyone to go on a violence spree, or as referred to earlier, that terrible mind are real or correct, but I do keep in mind that records the primitive thing humans capable of violence can skip a protracted way.

Scrupulosity and Religious OCD

We're going to want to mission out a bit on this segment as I am going to interrupt the unstated rule that I as a Western writer attempting to find out a scientific situation am not supposed to mention religion. This section is literary taboo because of the reality similar to the celebrated first-rate that church and country ought to be separate, church and treatment are also expected to be separate. Our felony tips restrict clinical doctors and clinical facilities from denying remedy because of non secular affiliation, so the ones caregivers have to live open and in the end silent close to religion. However, the fact is that OCD does now not care about our political correctness. Religion can play a large function within the state of affairs. It can be and regularly is flat out wrong about tremendous troubles and may make a contribution to highbrow distress.

I am not right here to trade every body's religious beliefs, so I will no longer circulate into element of the content material that I explored in some unspecified time in the future of my journey. For the sake of addressing a scientific scenario, however, I will address the concern factor because of the truth fear is what permits this subject matter to enhance to OCD.

As stated in advance, faith, especially monotheistic faith, threatens very excessive consequences for the untrue and might consequently generate large fear for devout enthusiasts who are induced take delivery of as proper with that they ought to be righteous in God's eyes, in any other case. Much of, if no longer all of this worry isn't realistic as maximum threats of punishment are every observe out of context or are borrowed from Pagan and special out of doors affects inside the first location.

The idea of hell as an everlasting area of torment did now not exist in the Old Testament. The lifeless wandered in an area referred to as "Sheol," which grow to be no longer in truth exquisite or terrible; it simply became. It come to be now not until the ones standards started performing within the likes of Persian, Greek and Chinese holy books that the idea of hell made its way into Judeo-Christian scripture, after which Islam took the danger of painful damnation to a trendy diploma.

In essence, this leaves us with possibilities: Either God did now not trouble revealing the doctrine of hell as an everlasting location of struggling until loads of years after He stimulated the Torah whilst close by pagan peers coincidentally superior similar thoughts brief previous, or, the sources collaborated and produced comparable messages at some point of the board that were uninspired, guy-made and must now not be feared. If we are able to appreciably keep in mind the second one possibility, this will lessen the concern of punishment that faith threatens.

In addition, it's miles appreciably arguable whether or not or not or now not the New Testament writers purported to painting hell as a physical region besides due to the fact the primary fear of first century Jews became to be stricken with the aid of shame in choice to from bodily pain. In Revelation, lack of lifestyles is said to be thrown into the Lake of Fire. This makes no experience functionally because of the fact demise isn't a bodily object, so certainly the descriptions of hell have been metaphoric to as a minimum a few degree. In Islamic scripture, the descriptions of hell within the Quran are sincerely terrifying and bodily, however the interpretation of the New Testament that Muhammad received inside the seventh century had already been altered.

Since worry is OCD's (and religion's) gasoline, lowering fear is critical. What we don't want to get up with non secular OCD is to get caught up in a entice of trying to out-assume our doubts via manner of locating solutions. OCD can by no means be beaten with the useful resource of manner of locating statistics. We can answer a question, but some different question will certainly appear thereafter. Since an obsessive thoughts will ask enough questions for five lifetimes, there's no manner to discover all of the answers in a single. Furthermore, we can doubt the solutions we find out besides! In the case of critical ideologies along side religion and politics, humans are going to in the long run take delivery of as true with what they need to trust. What we need to do in this situation then is release ourselves from the bondage of fear to permit ourselves the liberty to find the solutions that we're able to and amplify beliefs that we may be at peace with.

Relationship OCD

"When you discover the proper person, you may recognize it." "Find your soul mate." These expressions have come to be 2d nature to us. How lower priced are they despite the fact that? Perhaps a strong assessment may be made to the idealistic dream that everybody should do what they love for a living, which everyone recite to ourselves often on the cost of by no means finding contentment in our expert lives. It can occur for a pick out few, however operating in your dream profession isn't always the first-class manner to be happy and it is not mathematically possible for all people to do besides due to the reality then there will be no man or woman left to construct roads, clean lavatories and choose up trash. Society could not function. We all comprehend the infeasibility of such ideologies, but we hold close to them with all our also can. These useful mind moreover may be a luring and consuming lure for the obsessive thoughts.

The reality is that assignment delight is observed at the same time as we're obsessed with what we do, not continually even as we do what we're passionate about. Love does not continuously work within the real worldwide the way it does within the movies both. Perhaps every pornography for guys and romance novels and reality shows for women make contributions to those fantasies that location us so excessive on an imaginary hedonic treadmill that it is extraordinarily hard for a Westerner to discover contentment in a dating. What is possibly precise about this challenge count number is this war is experienced through using everyone at some point, and no longer sincerely via the use of way of OCD patients.

According to Isaac Newton's 1/3 law of motion, every pressure is located with the resource of way of an identical however opposite pressure. The international balances itself out in lots of procedures aside from in physics. Generally, the more ability a activity requires, the greater it's going to pay, and jobs that require less expertise pay an awful lot much less. The extra attractive a geographic area, the greater expensive it's far to live there, and the a great deal less appealing a geographic place, the loads a great deal much less steeply-priced it is. Higher exceptional meals is extra steeply-priced, tougher paintings outs are extra powerful, better diets require more issue, and lots of others.

If you pay interest, you could be aware how our universe has a totally constant and brilliant, but often times annoying manner of balancing itself out. Relationships and enchantment in favored art work very in addition. For instance, a person this is extra physical attractive and/or a hit may be greater in demand. They will consequently be a lot less appreciative in their friends and vice-versa. We have a supply and call for appraisal way for selecting pals that is basically time-honored and normal.

Searching for the perfect mate can end up an endless cycle of filling gaps from one accomplice to some different. At the surrender of the day, the amazing alternative is probably to put as much as the stability of the universe and apprehend that there may be usually a trade-off with relationships. Like an algebra equation with more than one avenues to remedy, there are numerous specific types of people we are in a position to connect to that may fulfill one in all a type dreams and make us glad in specific, however identical strategies. People often get caught in their very own slender system for the appropriate courting and restriction themselves to that container which now not frequently, if ever, suits precisely the way they need it to. Thus, those human beings never find out the happiness they may be searching out. Those who try to squeeze the arena into a place never escape that vicinity.

Now, this isn't always to say we must take shipping of certainly genuinely all and sundry or stay in an abusive or neglectful dating, however the countless search for the best mate in a global of stability and variety is not most effective unneeded, but it's miles a breeding floor for obsessive minds to conflict. We don't need to triumph over ourselves up over finding the right relationship, and we don't need to strain our partners to expose into the extraordinary companions. We can be happier than we ever knew we can be by way of studying to in reality receive our companions for who they're, information the balances and going for walks to beautify ourselves along the way.

Chapter 11: Homosexual Ocd

I am saving likely the most apparent distortion thru society and one of the most commonplace OCD struggles for remaining because of the truth that is the handiest that can actually start the reader down the course of understanding how our environments and located perceptions play a function in OCD. Sexual orientation is a absolutely not unusual motive for distress in lots of sufferers, and some of it is not desired.

Let's begin with the aid of manner of the usage of exploring why animals do not struggle with doubts over whether or not or not they are homosexual: The primary motive is due to the fact they do no longer have language to speak about their sexuality neither is there faith or a society influencing their expectations. Our ability to talk with verbal language is one of our most wonderful items that has enabled us to assemble knowledge technology upon technology. However, any incredible detail comes at a charge. In this situation, our language regularly labels and limitations our sexuality to 3 slender training: heterosexual, bisexual and gay even as truth paints a miles extra complicated photograph.

We label ourselves similarly in politics, however in politics, we have a 4-directional political compass which can plot one's political affairs everywhere among countless elements. No one is 100% conservative or one hundred% liberal, and no person is one hundred% authoritarian or one hundred% libertarian. Everyone falls somewhere within the middle of each axis. However, we regularly experience forced to label our political leanings as one way or the alternative the identical manner society expects us to label our sexuality one manner or the other.

Physically, every person starts offevolved out as lady until the exceptional chromosome makes 1/2 of folks male. This is why guys have nipples. Our our bodies are therefore not virtually superb. Our minds and what our eyes see aren't honestly one-of-a-type each. All men and all ladies can differentiate among an attractive and an unattractive member of the equal or opposite sex. Our genitalia are also not knowledgeable to react to first-rate the possibility intercourse, so it's miles bodily viable for all people to workout gay hobby, as do many individuals of the animal nation. Like our political opinions, our sexuality can unique itself in limitless approaches at some stage in a spectrum. While choosing a normal sexual conduct is truely an less high-priced choice that maximum humans make, which encompass myself, it is an injustice to obsessive doubters to sense forced to squeeze this choice into 3, or even instructions. These sufferers are trapped in a area that prevents them from manifestly viewing their sexuality as a complex, growing and evolving phenomenon.

Like each instance I've used, I am no longer suggesting that patients commonly act upon their doubts. The answer for HOCD patients isn't always constantly to adopt a completely specific sexual practice, but truely know-how and being at peace with their greater true nature and wherein those doubts originate from is more powerful than virtually denying them.

Chapter 12: What You Do No Longer Recognize Approximately Obsessive-Compulsive Ailment (Ocd)?

You had a busy day, and you decide to rest for the night time even as you do not forget that you could have left the the front door unlocked. You grow to be concerned and visit see if it's miles locked. Once you've checked that it's secured, you lighten up and pass lower returned to mattress. This not unusual tension is beneficial for you since it guarantees that you're vigilant about your surroundings.

Sometimes, although, those mind might be normal and evident. You may fit check the door and verify that it's steady, but whilst you pass once more to bed, you begin to fear about it all another time. You pass take a look at the door over again and move again to mattress, but your fear lingers. These persistent ideas, which make you experience uneasy all the time and have an impact to your ordinary lifestyles in the gadget, are known as obsessions.

Obsessions can variety; some human beings are enthusiastic about cleanliness and may fear that their palms are germ-infested no matter the truth that they cleansed them a lot much less than a minute inside the beyond.

People with OCD sense brilliant worry and distress. To soothe this tension, humans do several recurrent sports known as compulsions.

Compulsions offer short consolation to people laid low with OCD. In extreme conditions, the temptation to behavior such things time and again can notably forestall someone's regular lifestyles sports. When this repetitive recurrence of obsessions accompanied thru repulsive conduct continues to limit a person's capability to feature in each day life, it can be a case of OCD.

What are the symptoms of OCD?

AOCD may be identified with the useful resource of studying a person's obsessive behaviors. The maximum favored styles of signs and signs are:

Cleanliness: People who have a continual dread of infection; frequently wash their palms and smooth the house.

Order: Some human beings are preoccupied with symmetry and order. To ease their tension, they may be determined rearranging books and flatware or aligning rugs, pillows, and cushions frequently.

Hoarders: Hoarders are folks that locate it difficult to do away with a few detail. They accumulate vintage newspapers, garb, emails, and specific stuff for no obvious purpose.

Counting: Such human beings often rely their gadgets and extraordinary gadgets applied in normal lifestyles, along with the big form of stairs on a staircase or the numerous lighting fixtures in a corridor. If they lose take into account, they pass returned and begin once more.

Safety: Some human beings have unreasonable anxieties about safety; they are continuously checking if the doors and home windows are solid, whether the range has been switched off, and so on.

If you witness such conduct in any man or woman , you'll likely strive speakme to them and inspiring them to visit a intellectual health professional for remedy.

Chapter 13: How To Identify Ocd In Your Child.

Does your teen continuously want to rewrite, reread, or redo projects or artwork? Are they constantly looking for reassurance? Do they often be concerned about dust and germs? If so, your infant can be living with obsessive-compulsive illness, or OCD, a scenario impacting one in every hundred American children.

Parents also can apprehend signs and symptoms of OCD as truely a section their toddler goes via, however they're really indicators of OCD-related problems that might linger on into maturity, and regularly, physicians don't take a look at for them.

A teen with OCD usually indicates repetitious, farfetched, and unrealistic thoughts and behaviors. These sports regularly fall below a 4-symptom cluster, which includes:

Harm and protection troubles: Does your teenager fear approximately successfully locking and unlocking doors? Are they often involved about protection and potential robbers in the community?

Contamination and Cleaning Worries: Does your teen pressure over washing their arms well? Are they excessively fixated on dust and germs?

Symmetry and order: Does your infant insist on drawing within the lines or no longer stepping on cracks whilst taking walks? Do they stress garments looking and feeling "even" or retaining topics in tremendous order?

Magical wondering or superstitions: Is your teen extreme about unfortunate numbers, shades, unique phrases, sayings, or superstitions and pals them with catastrophes or "awful matters" that might occur?

"Most kids experience periodic obsessive mind or needs for sameness, together with seeking to concentrate their favored story take a look at within the same way, have clothes experience or look "definitely right," or feeling safest when they get prepared for bed in a specific order," Williams stated. "But if the ones kinds of issues hassle you or your toddler for a couple of hour a day, it is probably time to visit a consultant."

Diagnosing OCD

OCD hasn't deemed a scenario until it reasons certainly one of 3 things:

influences your teenager for brought than an hour an afternoon.

bothers them or makes them sad or uneasy.

interferes with own family (e.G., temper tantrums), motives distractions at university, or receives in the way of connections with pals.

As with many tension illnesses, it's predominant to address OCD as early as feasible. When OCD stays untreated, it may get more excessive and progress into despair.

Chapter 14: Causes Of Ocd In Youngsters.

Parents don't growth OCD of their children due to shortcomings in their parenting talents. OCD isn't advanced via the use of the way you interact together together with your children, don't talk with them, or the manner to area them. And it doesn't be counted variety whether or not or now not or not or no longer each parents work, there can be a live-at-home Mom or Dad, the dad and mom are divorced, or a determine remarries after divorce. Stress may additionally additionally furthermore make OCD worse in a baby already vulnerable to the ailment, however your moves didn't create the OCD.

What Doesn't Cause OCD

Brain Differences.

Using neuroimaging generation in which snap shots of the mind and its hobby are accumulated, researchers have been able to establish that positive regions of the thoughts paintings in some other manner in human beings with OCD as compared with those who don't. Research findings display that OCD signs and signs and symptoms and signs and symptoms also can entail conversation issues amongst numerous sections of the mind, collectively with the orbitofrontal cortex, the anterior cingulate cortex (each inside the the the front of the mind), the striatum, and the thalamus (deeper quantities of the mind). Abnormalities in neurotransmitter systems— materials like serotonin, dopamine, and glutamate (and probable others) that transfer indicators among mind cells—are also related to the condition.

The Gene Connection

Research financed through the National Institutes of Health studied DNA, and the results advocate that OCD and numerous comparable highbrow issues may be related with a very precise mutation of the human serotonin transporter gene (hSERT). People with severe OCD signs and symptoms can also have a 2d mutation in the same gene. Other research hint at a probable genetic issue as well.

About 25% of OCD patients have an immediate family member with the scenario. In addition, twin studies have indicated that if one dual has OCD, the alternative is much more likely to have it while the twins are equal, as opposed to fraternal. Overall, studies of twins with OCD suggest that inheritance contributes greater or much less forty five–sixty five% to the danger of having the sickness.

It's difficult to effectively estimate the possibilities that a discern will bypass OCD on (i.E., genetically) to his or her infant, no matter the truth that one of the mother and father has OCD or has a own family data of OCD. In maximum conditions, the probabilities are minimal that your youngsters may additionally moreover accumulate OCD. If you're a capability figure and have fears approximately whether or no longer or not your destiny kids can also furthermore inherit

OCD, it's sensible to speak about it along side your scientific doctor. Many maximum essential clinical facilities have genetic counselors on frame of personnel or with the useful resource of referral who may also additionally furthermore cope with this depend with you. The genetics of OCD is a subject of cutting-edge research, and breakthroughs come frequently.

Other Factors That May Contribute to the Onset of OCD

Several extra variables can also play a function in the formation of OCD, which includes behavioral, cognitive, and environmental problems. Learning theorists, as an instance, argue that behavioral schooling can also additionally additionally make contributions to the genesis and renovation of obsessions and compulsions. More precisely, they experience that compulsions are taught sports activities that help an individual decrease or cast off worry or pain associated with obsessions or urges.

An character who has an obsessive fixation on germs, as an instance, might also additionally take part in hand washing to alleviate the tension created through the obsession. Because this washing workout proper now soothes anxiety, the possibility that the individual could have interplay in hand washing while a infection worry takes area within the destiny is boosted. As a stop result, compulsive behavior no longer only maintains however becomes immoderate.

Many cognitive theorists declare that sufferers with OCD have faulty or dysfunctional beliefs and that it's far their misinterpretation of intrusive thoughts that motive the beginning area of obsessions and compulsions. According to the cognitive version of OCD, everybody reports intrusive mind. People with OCD, but, mistake the ones notions as being notably crucial, in my view great, revealing approximately one's character, or having devastating ramifications. The non-stop misinterpretation of undesired thoughts effects within the improvement of obsessions. Because the obsessions are so disturbing, the person engages in compulsive sports to try to fight, block, or neutralize them.

The Obsessive-Compulsive Cognitions Working Organization, an global company of teachers who have hypothesized that the onset and maintenance of OCD are associated with maladaptive interpretations of cognitive intrusions, has diagnosed six categories of dysfunctional beliefs associated with OCD:

Inflated duty: a sense that one may additionally purpose and/or is answerable for preventing unwanted situations;

Importance of thoughts (furthermore known as "concept-movement fusion"): the belief that having a horrible belief should boom the threat of the superiority of a negative occasion or that having horrible questioning (e.G., considering performing some aspect) is morally much like doing it;

Control of thoughts: A notion that it is each vital and possible to have wellknown manipulate over one's questioning;

Overestimation of threat: a belief that terrible occurrences are extremely feasible and that they might be quite painful;

Perfectionism: the concept that one cannot make errors and that imperfection is terrible; and

Intolerance for uncertainty: a perception that it's far critical and possible to apprehend, certainly, that terrible occurrences received't seem.

Environmental events may also furthermore contribute to the onset of OCD. For example, severe mind injuries had been related to the formation of OCD, which gives additional evidence of a linkage between mind feature impairment and OCD.

Sudden onset of OCD signs and symptoms.

Some dad and mom have said that OCD signs and symptoms arose absolutely in a single day as although a switch have been have grow to be; their youngster went to bed as the child they knew and wakened a stranger. For some years, this speedy start of signs and symptoms and symptoms and symptoms has been taken into consideration to upward thrust up in mixture with a strep contamination, which initiates OCD and/or tic signs and signs in children who're genetically liable to the sickness. This kind of unexpected-onset OCD grew to grow to be identified as Pediatric Autoimmune Neuropsychiatric Disorders Associated with Streptococcal Infections, or PANDAS.

In the greater recent beyond, researchers and clinicians have confirmed that regardless of the fact that strep may be a cause for OCD, it is able to not be the most effective cause. Non-strep ailments at the side of Lyme illness, mononucleosis, and the flu virus (e.G., H1N1) can also create identical intellectual troubles in sensitive kids. As a surrender cease result, specialists have up to date the name of the illness to Pediatric Acute-Onset Neuropsychiatric Syndrome, or PANS. The vital standards for PANS are

(1) an abrupt and dramatic onset of OCD signs and signs and symptoms that is associated with brilliant impairment, and

(2) the simultaneous, speedy onset of various signs and symptoms from as a minimum two of 7 commands: anxiety, emotional instability, and/or melancholy; irritability, aggression, and/or oppositional behaviors; behavioral regression; sudden deterioration in college usual performance; sensory or motor abnormalities, mainly handwriting issues; and somatic, or bodily, symptoms and signs and signs and symptoms and signs and symptoms.

Currently, PANDAS and PANS are significantly underneath-researched. Until the time that appropriate remedy centered especially at PANS is available, treatments traditionally applied within the remedy of PANDAS (e.G., antibacterial drugs, publicity and reaction prevention, selective serotonin reuptake inhibitors) can be useful, depending upon the man or woman desires of the child.

Chapter 15: What Are The Signs Of Ocd And Their Influence On Children?

The symptoms and signs and symptoms of OCD consist of each obsessive and compulsive sports.

Signs of obsession encompass:

Repeated unwanted mind.

Fear of infection.

Aggressive impulses.

Persistent sexual thoughts.

Images of hurting a person you want or mind that you could inflict harm on someone.

Thoughts that you will be damage.

Signs of compulsion include:

Constant checking.

Constant counting.

The regular washing of one or more topics.

Repeatedly cleansing your palms.

Constantly checking the range or door locks.

Arranging items to face a specific way.

Emotional Symptoms of Obsessive-Compulsive Disorder.

Sufferers of OCD are often as a substitute involved and emotional. They display numerous non-OCD signs and symptoms and symptoms, which includes signs and signs of sadness, immoderate venture, excessive anxiety, and the chronic sensation that now not whatever is ever right.

Physical Symptoms of Obsessive-Compulsive Disorder.

Aside from the apparent obsessive behaviors someone with OCD suggests, there aren't any physical caution signs of this situation; yet, someone with OCD ought to in all likelihood growth clinical problems. For instance, someone with a germ preoccupation also can furthermore wash their fingers so frequently that the pores and skin on them gets pink, raw, and uncomfortable.

Short-Term and Long-Term Effects of OCD.

A character with OCD also can face many short-term affects, covered in the lack of capacity to carry out as a contributing member of society, disturbing conditions at university or paintings, or problems preserving friendships or love relationships. The prolonged-term repercussions of OCD often upward push up due to the low excellent of life that maximum severe sufferers have. Long-time period impacts include sadness, continual worry, and an advanced threat of substance dependence.

It is recommended to embark at the route to healing as speedy as feasible to prevent the worsening of those outcomes. Give us a name on our helpline in recent times.

Is there a check or self-evaluation I can do?

If your circle of relatives have informed you that you have obsessive mind or are compulsive in movement, you've got simply realized that you do have sure compulsive inclinations. Most humans with OCD are aware of the movements they may be appearing; they simply can't save you them.

There is not any self-assessment exam for OCD sufferers, but you may self-affirm by getting together together with your family and growing with a list of behaviors you continuously show. You can then communicate this listing together together together with your healthcare organization.

After speaking to you approximately your ideals and habits, your physician also can prescribe a intellectual examination. Your physician might also additionally moreover want to talk in your family and close to pals.

Chapter 16: How Is Ocd Treated?

Treatment can be specifically useful for youngsters with OCD, supporting them to enjoy complete and productive lives.

A certified highbrow health professional is excellent suitable to deal with pediatric OCD the usage of a form of cognitive conduct remedy (CBT) called exposure and response prevention (ERP).

In ERP, youngsters learn how to face their troubles (publicity) without giving in to compulsions (response prevention). A licensed highbrow health practitioner (inclusive of a psychologist, social worker, or counselor) will teach them through this way, and youngsters will research that they will allow their obsessions and anxieties come and bypass with out the need for his or her compulsions or rituals. Click proper here for help deciding on the great therapist to your infant or teen. Psychiatric medicine can be explored if the kid's signs and signs and symptoms are very intense and/or not alleviated with the aid of the usage of ERP on my own.

A particular form of antidepressant referred to as serotonin reuptake inhibitors (SRIs) has been established to noticeably lessen OCD signs and signs and symptoms and symptoms in children and young adults, making ERP much less complicated to behavior and greater a success.

Medications must best be supplied via a licensed clinical expert (which incorporates your pediatrician or a psychiatrist) who has experience operating with children and teenagers and can ideally artwork together collectively together with your therapist to build a treatment plan. Click proper proper right here to observe greater approximately pills for OCD in kids and young adults. When combined, ERP and remedy are regarded due to the fact the "first-line" remedies for OCD. Start proper here, in one-of-a-kind terms! About 70 percent of sufferers will advantage from ERP and/or medication for his or her OCD.

Family Involvement OCD can be quite preserving aside and is specific in that obsessions and rituals can every now and then include individuals of the family. Parents and caregivers (or maybe siblings every now and then) are a important element of a baby's OCD treatment and should be involved in severa processes. Click right proper here to discover extra about resources for households.

Other remedy alternatives Support corporations can also be useful for kids and teens with OCD, as well as their own family contributors. Support businesses provide the functionality to connect and take a look at from other individuals who recognize what they're going through. There are even a few manual agencies exclusively for dad and mom of youngsters with OCD.

If your baby or teen has engaged in normal outpatient remedy (seeing a therapist 1-2 times constant with week in their place of work) and would love to strive a greater huge diploma of care, there are greater possibilities. The IOCDF maintains a useful useful resource list of extensive remedy facilities, expert outpatient packages, and therapists that provide severa ranges of remedy for OCD in children and teens. The following lists of healing options are from least tremendous to maximum intensive:

Traditional outpatient. Patients meet a therapist for person durations as often as indicated by manner of way of their therapist, regularly one or instances consistent with week for 45–50 mins. (Most therapists within the Resource Directory, similarly to many "strong factor outpatient clinics," provide this form of remedy).Intensive outpatient. Patients might also attend businesses and one character session in line with day, multiple days in keeping with week.

Clinics labeled as "intensive treatment programs" within the Resource Directory provide this diploma of treatment. Day utility. Patients go through treatment at a few degree in the day (frequently corporation and character treatment) at a mental health remedy middle, typically from nine a.M. To 5 p.M. Up to five days each week. Many centers categorized as "in depth remedy programs" in the Resource Directory provide this degree of remedy. Partial hospitalization. Same due to the fact the day application, besides humans attend therapy at a highbrow health group.

Several centers categorized as "incredible remedy applications" inside the Resource Directory provide this diploma of treatment. Residential. Patients are treated whilst dwelling willingly in an unlocked intellectual health treatment center or clinic. Clinics classified as "residential" inside the Resource Directory offer this diploma of remedy. Inpatient. This is the best degree of contend with a intellectual health ailment.

Treatment is brought in a limited putting at a intellectual clinic on a voluntary or on occasion involuntary basis. Patients are admitted to this degree of care if they are no longer succesful to attend to themselves or are a risk to themselves or others. Inpatient remedy pursuits to stabilize the affected character, which commonly takes severa days to every week, and then pass the affected person to a decrease level of care. Other alternatives: Summer applications and camps Many rigorous remedy facilities now offer summer time "camps" for youngsters and teens with OCD.

These programs range in method and fashion, but maximum are form of in keeping with week prolonged and variety from traditional "sleep-away" camps to daylight hours camps wherein kids sleep at home or stay with loved ones close by. Click here to examine more.

What about PANDAS or PANS?

There is an superb type of OCD that starts in kids, simply as indicated above, following the immune tool's reactivity to an infection such as strep throat, causing rapid onset (apparently in a single day) OCD signs and symptoms and signs.

This shape of OCD is called Pediatric Autoimmune Neuropsychiatric Disorder Associated with Streptococcus (PANDAS) if it's miles a strep contamination or Pediatric Acute-Onset Neuropsychiatric Syndrome (PANS) if it's far any other contamination.

Children with PANDAS/PANS need to despite the reality that get ERP from a equipped mental health practitioner, but they will moreover want antibiotic remedy from their physician.

www.ingramcontent.com/pod-product-compliance
Lightning Source LLC
Chambersburg PA
CBHW060222030426
42335CB00014B/1306